AF890425

PHYSEO

TABLE OF CONTENTS

We would like to extend a special thanks to the following individuals who have spent many hours tutoring, guiding and consulting this work, making Physeo Anatomy possible.

David A. Morton, Ph.D.
Professor
Vice-Chair of Medical and Dental Education
Department of Neurobiology and Anatomy
University of Utah School of Medicine
Salt Lake City, UT

Julie Anne Jahp
MD Candidate, Class of 2022
University of Utah School of Medicine

Julie A. Hansen
Class of 2022
St. George's University SOM

CARDIOVASCULAR ANATOMY

Section I - Arteries of the Upper Body

I. There are seven arteries of the upper body that are important to know for board examinations. (See Table 3.1.1 - Upper body arteries)

Vessel	Anatomy	Notes
Subclavian artery	• From aortic arch (left side) • From brachiocephalic artery (right side)	• Subclavian steal (proximal stenosis → retrograde vertebral artery flow)
Intercostal arteries	• Anterior arteries arise from subclavian • Posterior arteries arise from aorta	• Rib notching in aortic coarctation
Internal carotid artery	• Supplies brain	• Involved in strokes
External carotid artery	• Supplies face, neck and nose (mostly via maxillary artery)	• Involved in face, neck or nose pathology • Epistaxis (especially medial nose) • Epidural hematoma (middle meningeal artery)
Brachial artery	• From axillary artery	• Damaged in distal humeral fractures with *median* nerve • Memory hook: "*Brake* before you hit the *median*, or you will be in *deep red* blood"
Deep brachial artery	• From brachial artery	• Damaged in mid-humeral fractures with radial nerve • Memory hook: "Brake before you hit the median, or you will be in deep red blood"
Radial artery	• From brachial artery • Branches into dorsal scaphoid branch	• Scaphoid fractures can result in proximal scaphoid bone necrosis

Table 3.1.1 - Upper body arteries

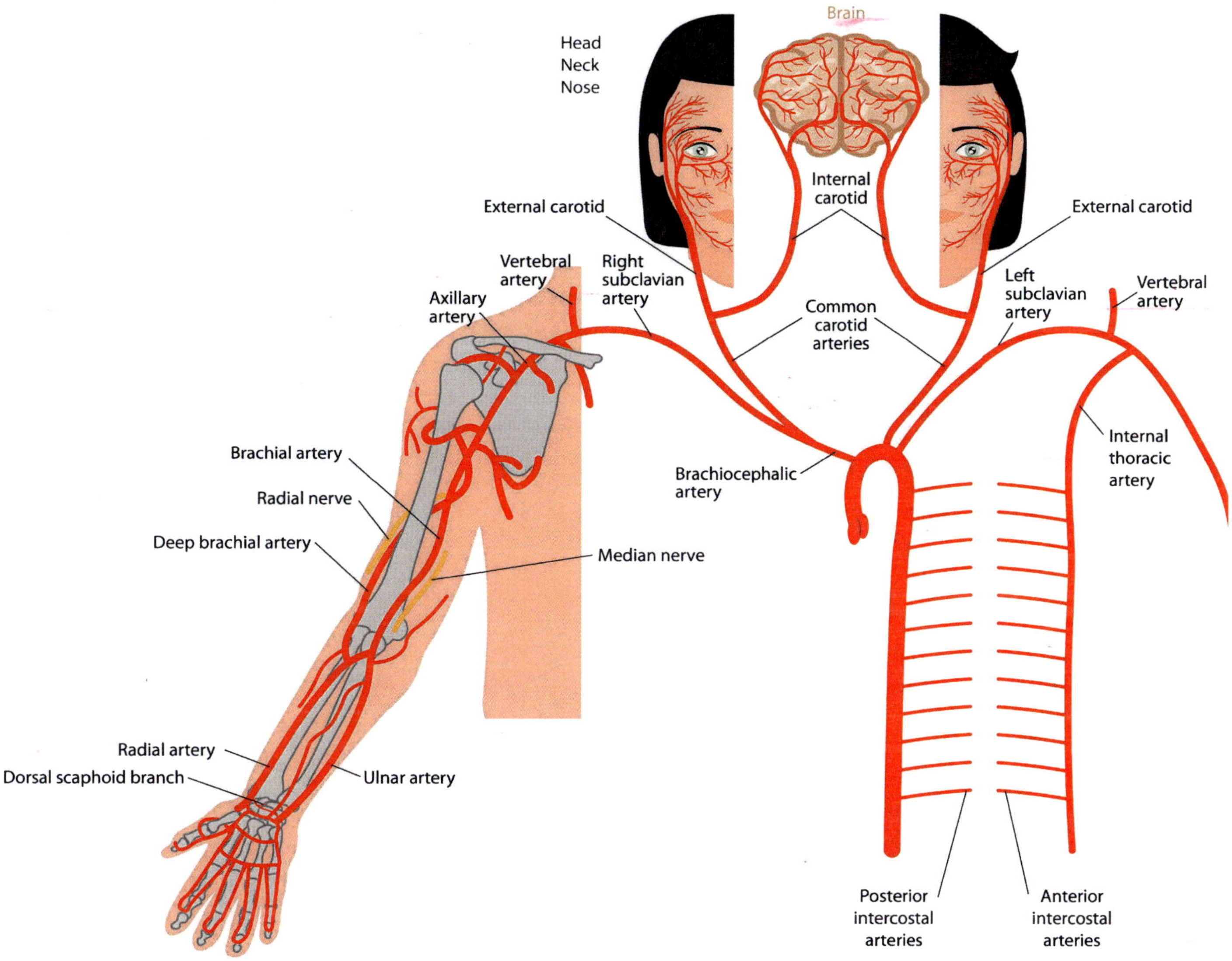

Figure 3.1.1 - Upper body arteries

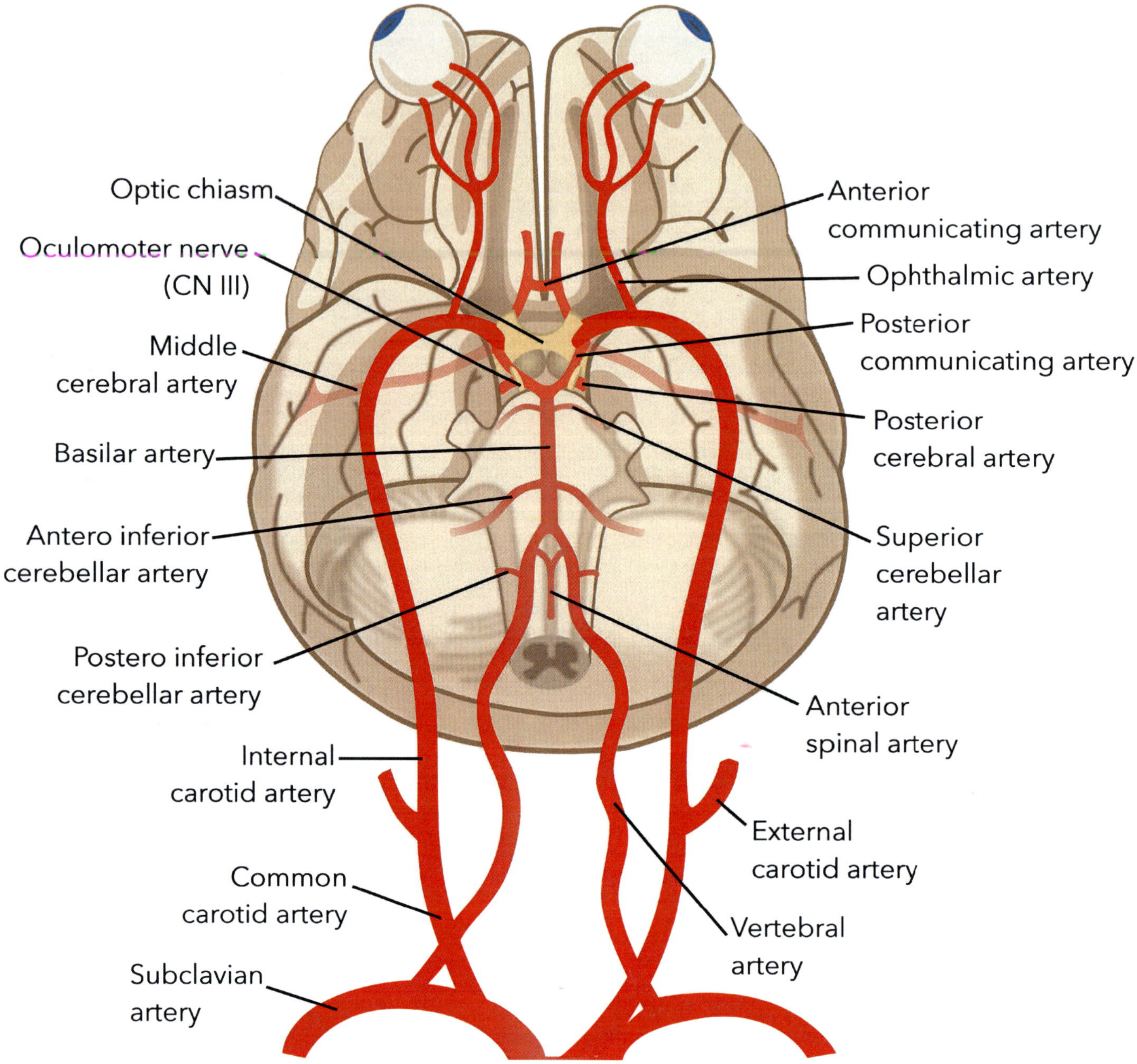

Figure 3.1.2 - Neurovasculature diagram

II. Subclavian Steal Syndrome

A. Proximal subclavian artery stenosis → increased pressure (decreased flow) in the vertebral artery on the same side as the obstruction → retrograde blood flow down the vertebral artery on the opposite side of the obstruction

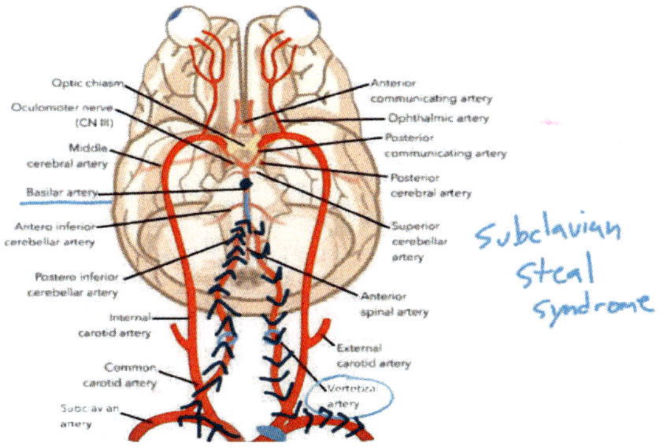

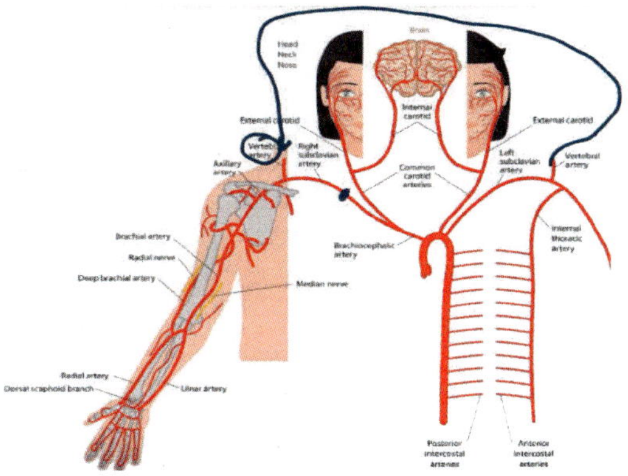

III. Aortic Coarctation

A. A narrowing of the descending aorta

1. Decreased flow to posterior intercostal arteries

2. Anterior intercostal arteries supply the posterior intercostals -Posterior intercostals engorge and damage inferior ribs over time (rib notching)

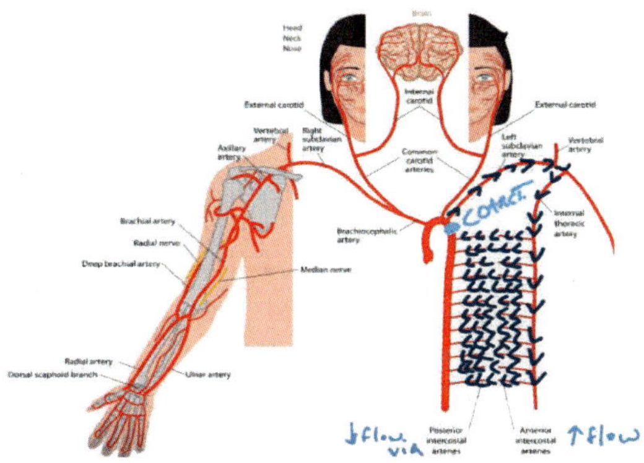

IV. Proximal scaphoid bone necrosis

A. The dorsal scaphoid branch from the radial artery provides blood to the distal portion of the scaphoid bone before traveling more proximally to supply the proximal scaphoid bone.

B. Fractures to the scaphoid bone can leave the distal portion well perfused, but the proximal portion without adequate oxygenation → necrosis

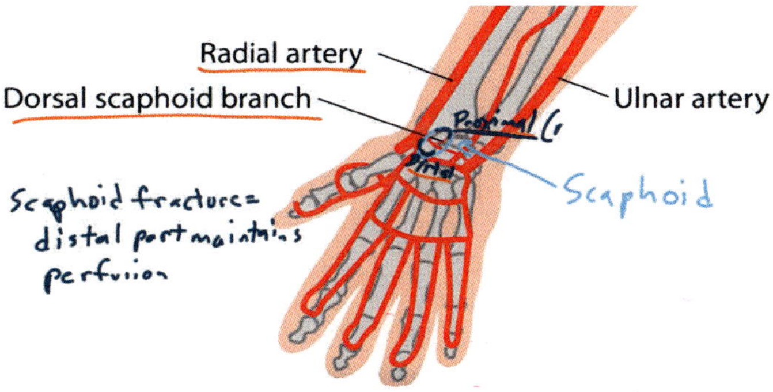

REVIEW QUESTIONS

?

1. A 30-year-old male presents to the emergency department following trauma to the nose during a snowboarding accident. Physical exam reveals profuse nasal bleeding. The damaged arteries resulting in this presentation originate from what vessel?

   A) Internal carotid artery
   B) External carotid artery
   C) Vertebral artery
   D) Middle meningeal artery
   E) Distal subclavian artery

- **Answer: Arteries in the face, neck and nose come from the maxillary artery, which is a branch of the external carotid artery.**
- **Most of the bleeding seen in this patient is likely from the medial nose, the nasal septum, where the vascular density is greatest**

2. An elderly patient is found to have vertebrobasilar insufficiency, resulting in frequent syncopal episodes. Extensive diagnostic evaluation reveals retrograde blood flow through the right vertebral artery directly into a major vessel. This major vessel arises directly from what artery?

- **Because this patient has retrograde blood flow through the right vertebral artery, we know this patient has subclavian steal syndrome.**
- **The "major vessel" receiving the blood from the right vertebral artery is the right subclavian artery, which arises directly from the brachiocephalic artery.**

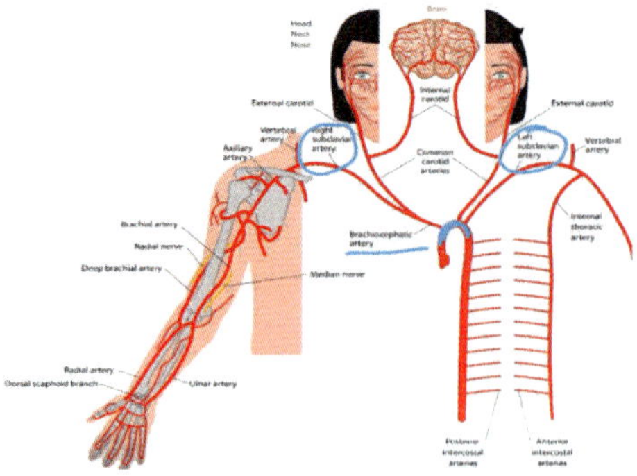

3. A 15-year-old boy is involved in a car accident and presents to the emergency department with profuse bleeding from his left arm. He is also unable to extend his wrist. A radiograph of the injured arm is obtained. Which artery is more likely damaged, the brachial, deep brachial or radial artery? What nerve is likely damaged?

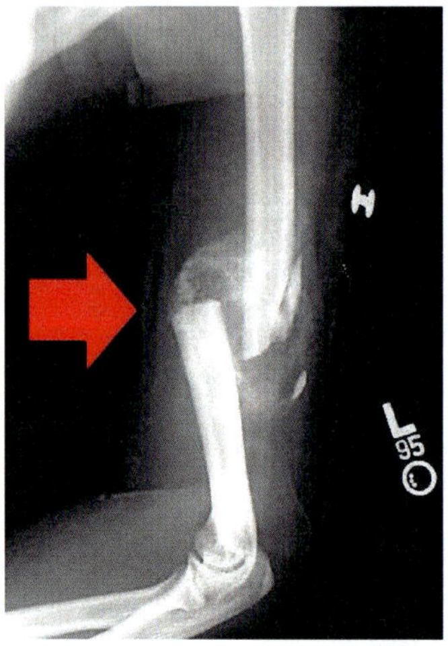

- **This image demonstrates a humerus with a midshaft fracture, which places the deep brachial artery in jeopardy. The deep brachial artery branches off the brachial artery and crosses the mid humerus in this midshaft region.**
- **The nerve often damaged with deep brachial artery injury is the radial nerve.**
- **Remember the memory hook: Brake before you hit the median, or you will be deep in red blood.**
- **Meaning that when you damage the deep brachial artery, you are also likely to damage the radial nerve at the same time.**
- **Or you could suspect radial nerve damage from the physical exam. We are told he cannot extend his wrist, which may tell you right there that he has radial nerve damage**

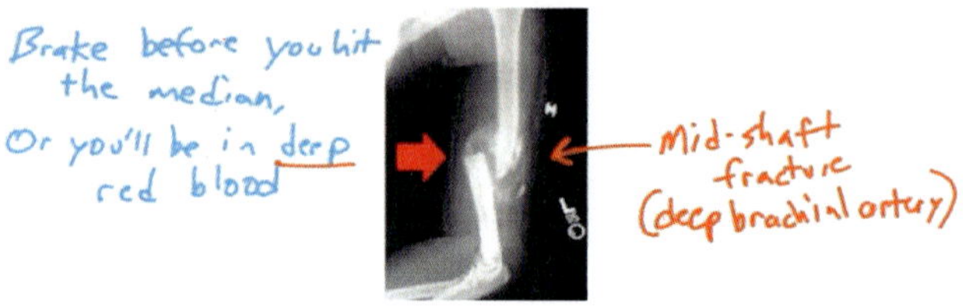

Section II - Veins of the Upper Body

I. There are primarily two major groups of veins that are important to know for board examinations. (See Table 3.1.2 - Upper body veins)

Vessel	Anatomy	Notes
Brachiocephalic veins	• Drain subclavian and internal jugular veins (IJV) • External jugular vein (EJV) drains into subclavian	• Obstruction causes unilateral swelling of tissues drained by EJV and subclavian • EJV drains the face and neck • IJV drains the brain
Superior vena cava (SVC)	• Drains right and left brachiocephalic veins • Returns blood to the right atrium	• Obstruction causes bilateral swelling (SVC syndrome) of tissues drained by EJV and subclavian

Table 3.1.2 - Upper body veins

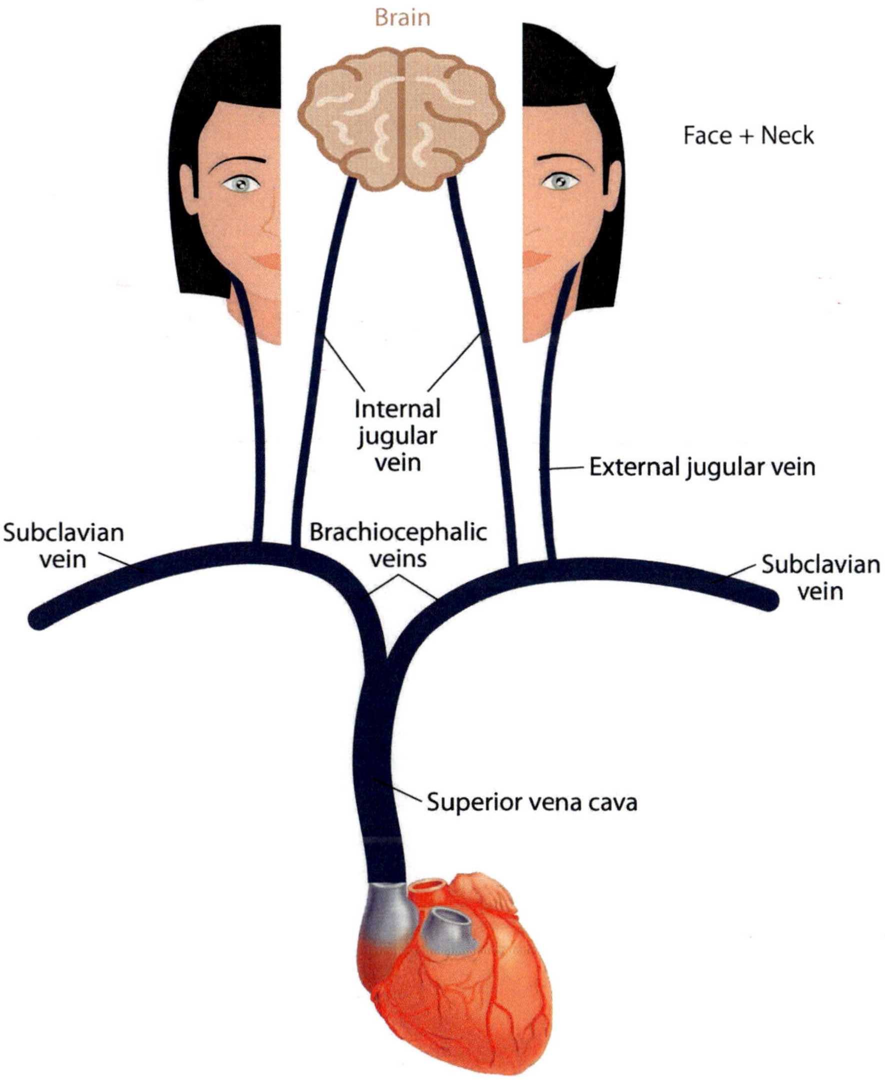

Figure 3.1.3 - Upper body veins

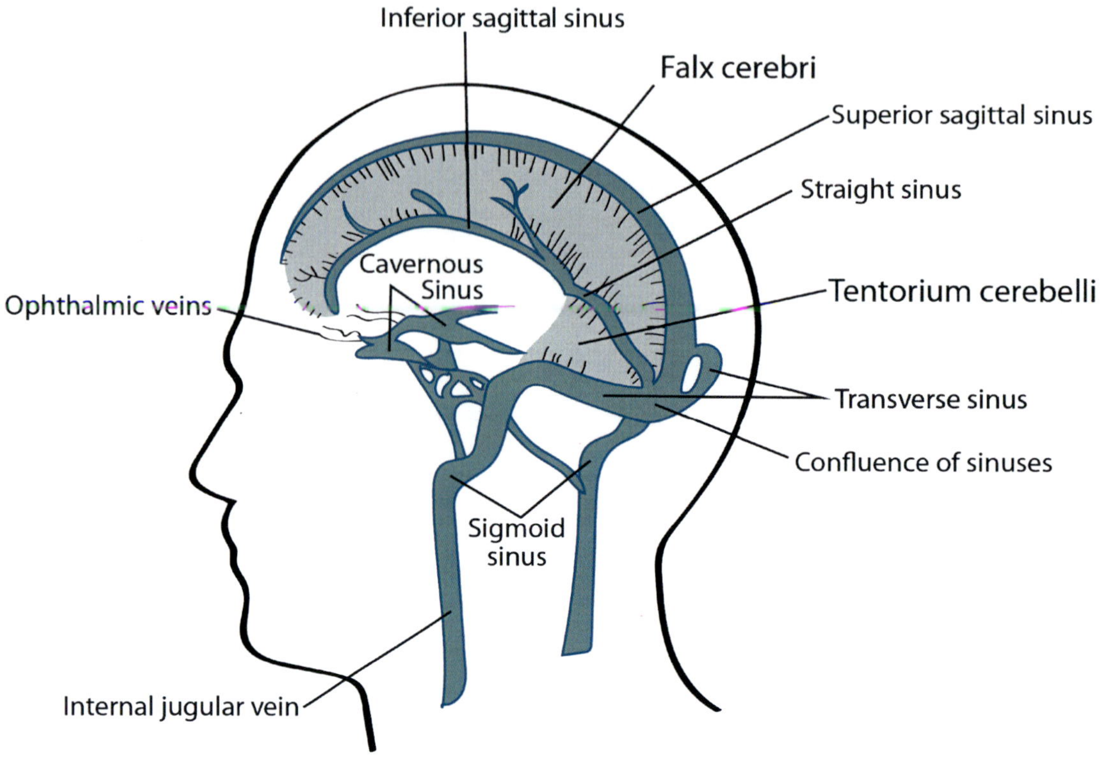

Figure 3.1.4 - Dural venous sinuses

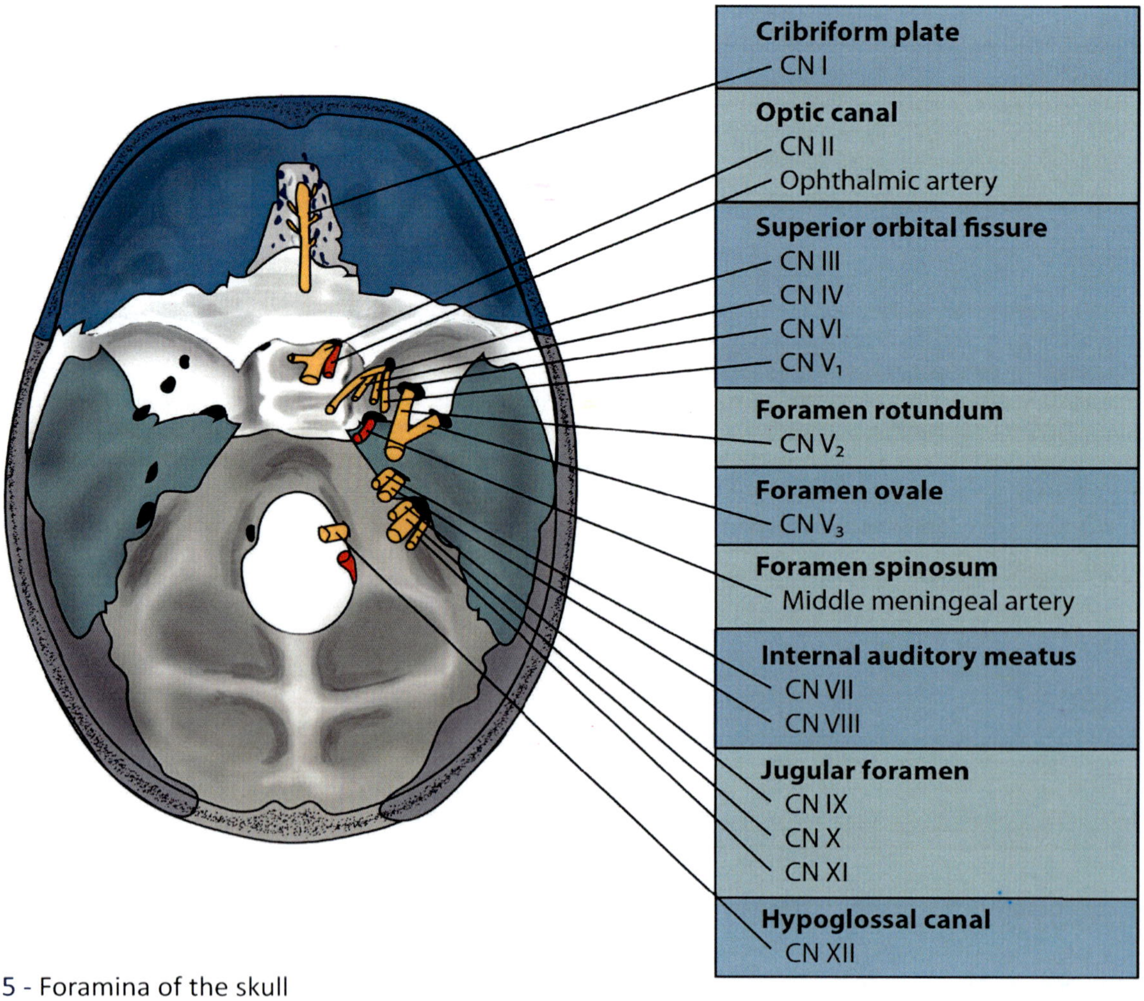

Figure 3.1.5 - Foramina of the skull

II. Internal jugular veins and internal carotid arteries supply the brain.

III. External jugular veins and the external carotid arteries supply the face and neck.

IV. Brachiocephalic vein obstruction

A. Obstruction of either brachiocephalic vein will cause *unilateral* swelling of the tissues drained by the external jugular vein (face and neck) and the subclavian vein (arm).

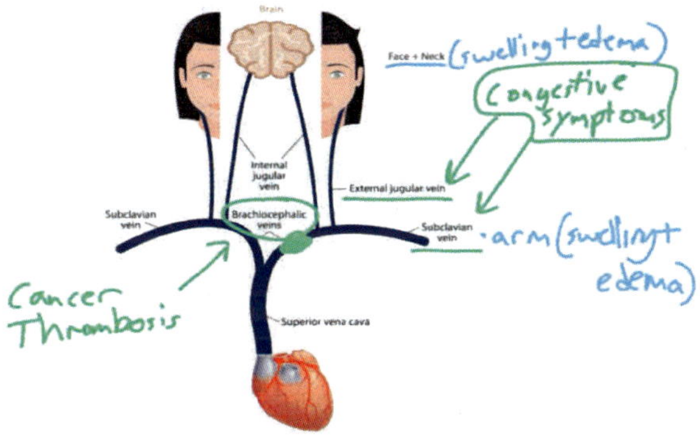

I. Superior vena cava obstruction (SVC)

A. Obstruction of the SVC will lead to *bilateral* congestion of tissues drained by the external jugular veins and the subclavian veins.

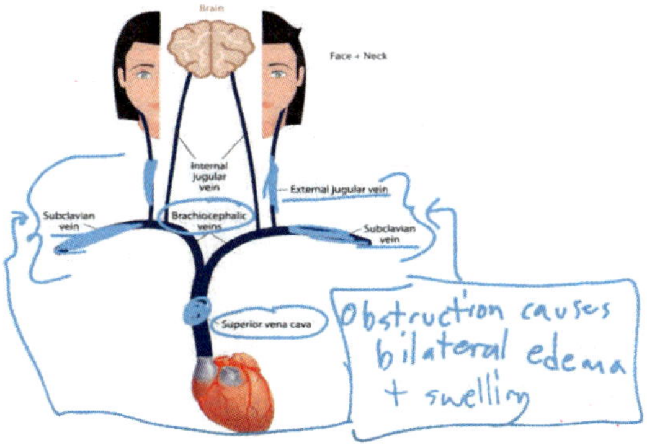

REVIEW QUESTIONS

1. A 73-year-old woman with a 43-pack-year history presents with coughing accompanied by bloody sputum for 3 months. A chest radiograph is obtained, indicating likely lung cancer. Physical exam reveals noticeable neck distension, a ruddy appearance and edematous hands. If the physical exam findings are caused by the mass seen on the radiograph, what vessel is directly involved?

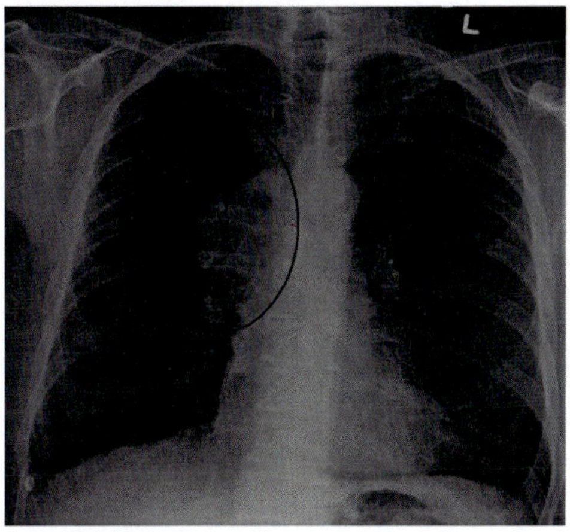

By James Heilman, MD [CC BY-SA 3.0 (https://creativecommons.org/licenses/by-sa/3.0) or GFDL (http://www.gnu.org/copyleft/fdl.html)], from Wikimedia Commons

A) Right brachiocephalic vein
B) Superior vena cava
C) Left brachiocephalic vein
D) Right external jugular vein
E) Left subclavian vein

- **Answer: The question stem states the hands (plural) are edematous. This should make you think of bilateral swelling. Only obstruction of the SVC, choice B, would lead to bilateral swelling.**
  - **Choices A, C, D and E indicate structures that are congested, but are not *directly* obstructed, so these choices are incorrect.**

Section III - Arteries of the Lower Body

I. There are five major groups of lower body arteries that are important to know for board examinations. (See Table 3.1.3 - Arteries of the lower body)

Vessel	Anatomy	Clinical Significance
Internal iliac artery	• Supplies uterine and vaginal arteries	• Ligate uterine artery in case of uterine hemorrhage
Inferior epigastric artery	• Branch of external iliac artery • Supplies abdominal wall below umbilicus	• Can be damaged during laparoscopic surgery
Femoral artery	• Distal to inguinal ligament	• Palpate pulse
Superficial epigastric artery	• Branch of femoral artery • Supplies superficial portion of abdominal wall below umbilicus	• Can be damaged during laparoscopic surgery
Medial circumflex artery	• Deep femoral artery (branch of femoral artery)	• Osteonecrosis of femoral head

Table 3.1.3 - Arteries of the lower body

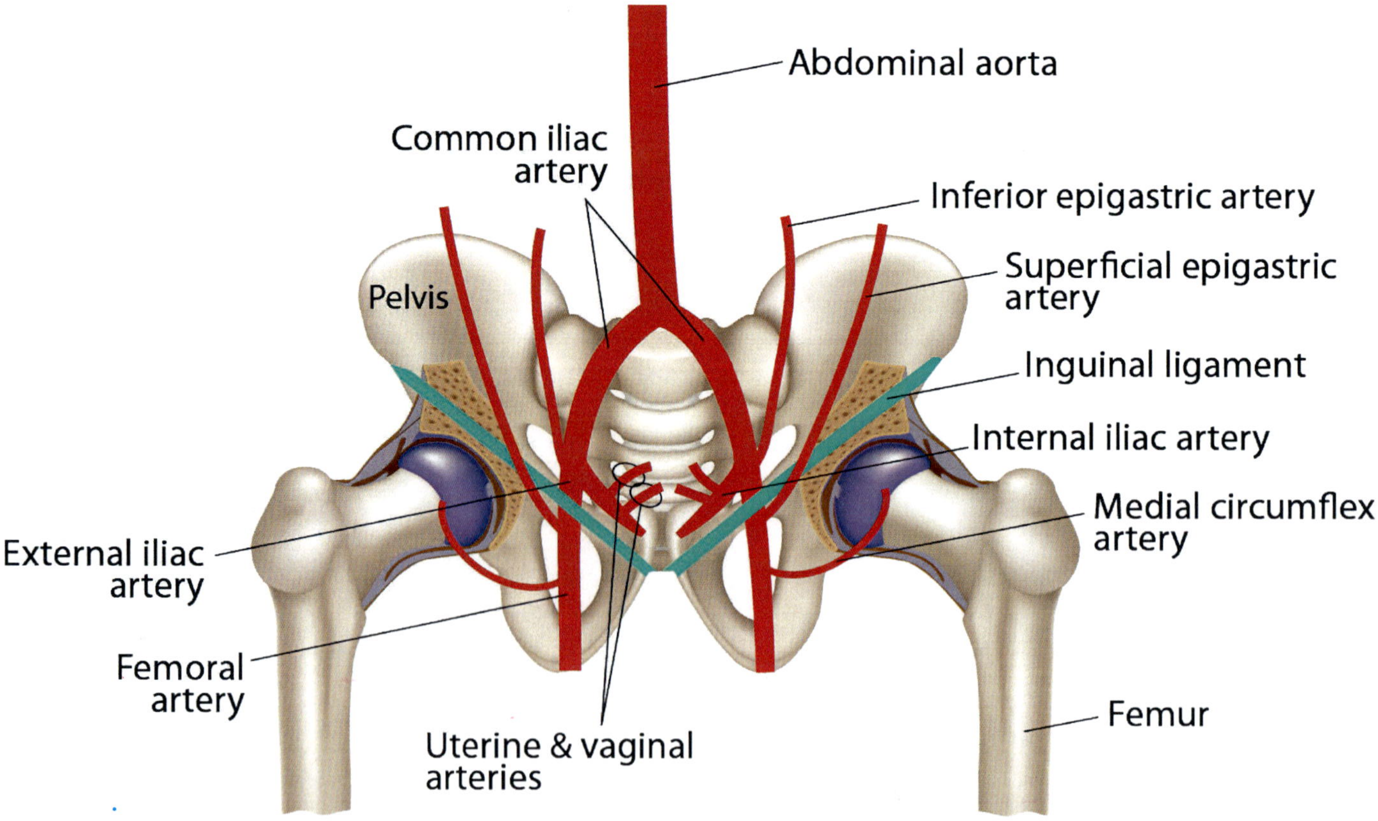

Figure 3.1.6 - Arteries of the lower body

REVIEW QUESTIONS

1. A 23-year-old man is involved in a motor vehicle accident. The medial circumflex artery is damaged, leading to osteonecrosis. Does this vessel originate above or below the inguinal ligament?

    - **Answer: Recall that the medial circumflex artery comes from the femoral artery, which is BELOW the inguinal ligament.**
    - **Notice that the common iliac splits into the internal iliac artery and the external iliac artery. Once the external iliac artery crosses the inguinal ligament, it becomes the femoral artery. The medial circumflex originates from the deep femoral artery, which is a branch of the femoral artery, which is BELOW the inguinal ligament.**

2. A 46-year-old female presents to the emergency department following a factory accident while working. During the accident the patient's right internal iliac artery was severely damaged. Further evaluation reveals that this was the only vessel damaged during the accident. Based upon the information above, which of the following structures will receive decreased blood flow?

    A) Femoral head
    B) Vagina
    C) Gastrocnemius muscle
    D) Lower abdominal wall

    - **Answer: The question was really asking, what structure receives blood from the internal iliac artery (the severely damaged vessel). The important structures supplied by the internal iliac artery include the uterus and the vagina. With severe damage to her *right* internal iliac artery, her uterus and vagina will be affected.**
        - **So the answer is B**
    - **The femoral head (choice A) is mainly supplied by the medial circumflex artery, ultimately deriving from the femoral artery.**
    - **The gastrocnemius muscle (choice C) is in the lower leg, which is ultimately supplied by the femoral artery.**
    - **And the lower abdomen (choice D) receives blood from the superficial epigastric artery, a branch of the femoral artery, as well as the inferior epigastric artery, a branch of the *external* iliac artery**

Section IV - Veins of the Lower Body

I. There are six major lower body veins that are important to know for board examinations. (See Table 3.1.4 - Lower body veins)

Vessel	Anatomy	Clinical Significance
Internal pudendal veins	• Empties into the internal iliac veins	• Plexus drains prostate, vulva, penis, and inferior rectum
Inferior rectal veins	• Drains rectum below pectinate line	• External and painful hemorrhoids • Anorectal varices in cirrhosis (anastomosis with superior rectal vein)
Vertebral venous plexus	• Drains vertebral bodies of spinal column • Communicates with internal iliac veins	• Cancers from pelvis can seed to vertebral bodies
Femoral vein	• Popliteal vein becomes femoral vein at adductor hiatus (adductor magnus) • Drains great saphenous vein • Drains superficial epigastric vein	• Deep vein thrombosis • Site of central venous line insertion
Great saphenous vein	• Drains into femoral vein at femoral triangle	• Superficial vein thrombosis • Cardiac grafts
Superficial epigastric vein	• Drains superficial abdominal wall	• Caput medusae in portal hypertension (anastomosis with paraumbilical veins)

Table 3.1.4 - Lower body veins

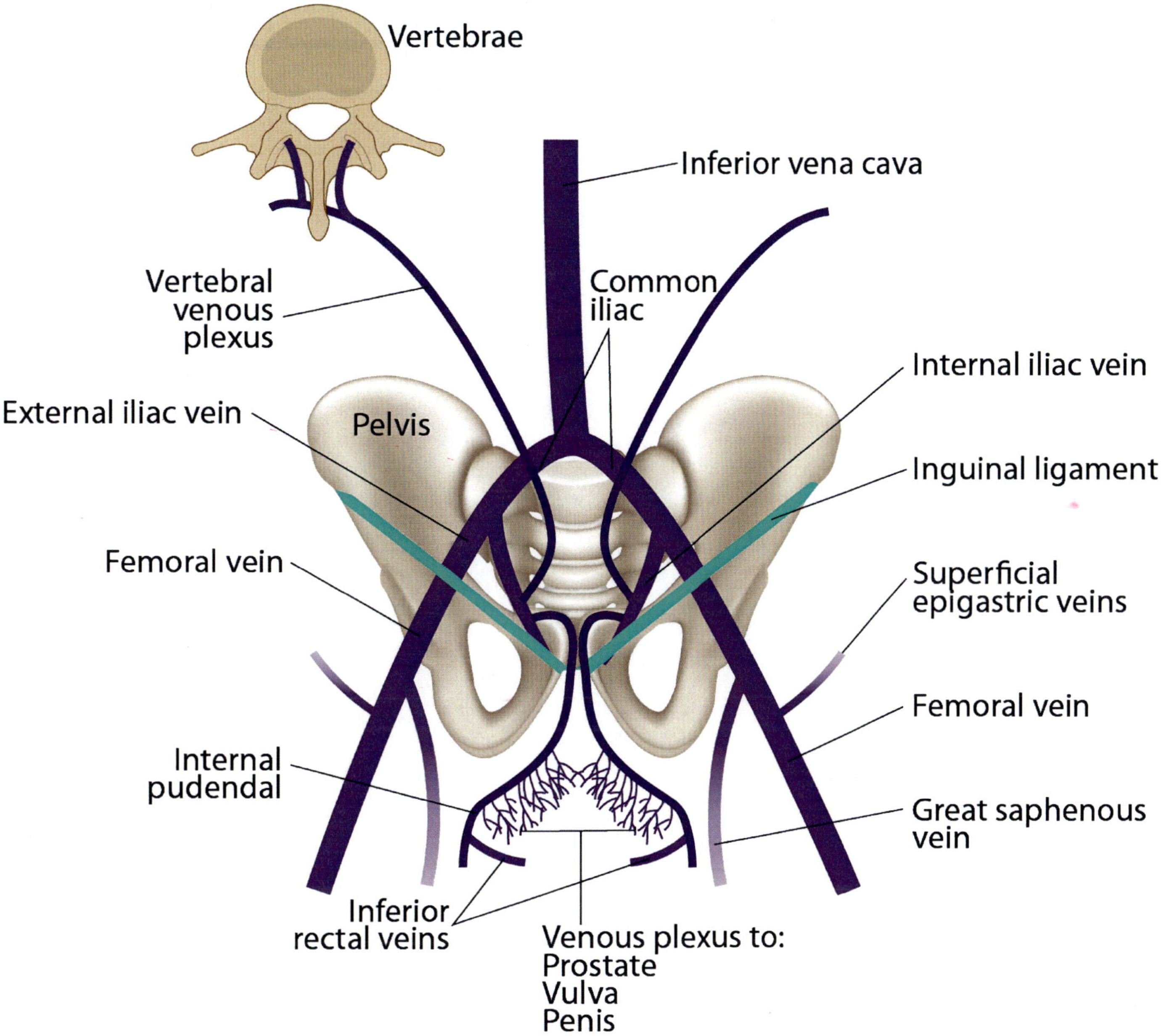

Figure 3.1.7 - Veins of the lower body

II. Hemorrhoids in the Context of Lower Body Veins

A. Hemorrhoids above the pectinate line are drained by the superior rectal veins.

B. Hemorrhoids below the pectinate line are drained by the inferior rectal veins.

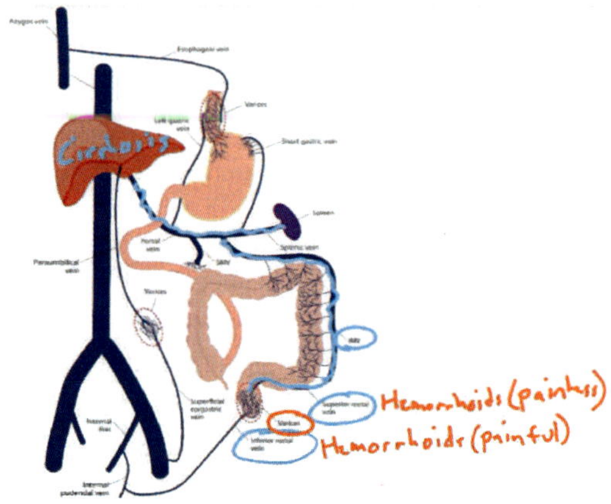

III. Vertebral Venous Plexus

A. Pelvic cancers (e.g. prostate cancers) can metastasize to the vertebral bodies by traveling through the vertebral venous plexus.

1. The vertebral venous plexus is valveless and bidirectional, allowing metastases to flow to the spine.

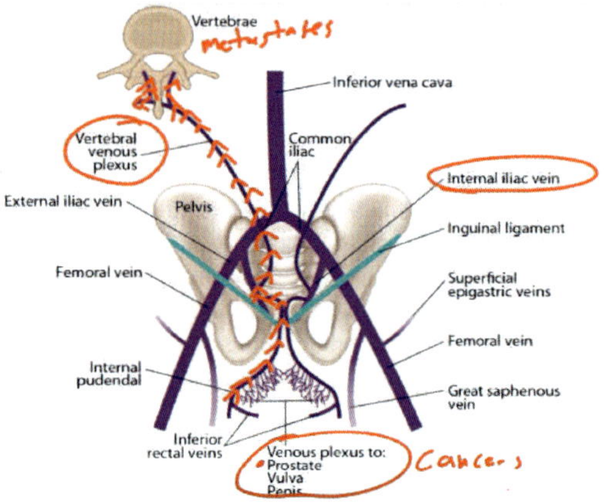

IV. Femoral Artery

A. Veins that drain the deep structures of the leg (popliteal vein and femoral vein) are considered deep. This means they can be the site of deep vein thromboses.

B. The great saphenous vein, is superficial and can be the site of superficial venous thromboses. The great saphenous vein is also useful for vascular grafts because it is superficial, it has moderate diameter, and is not crucial to the deep musculature of the leg and thigh.

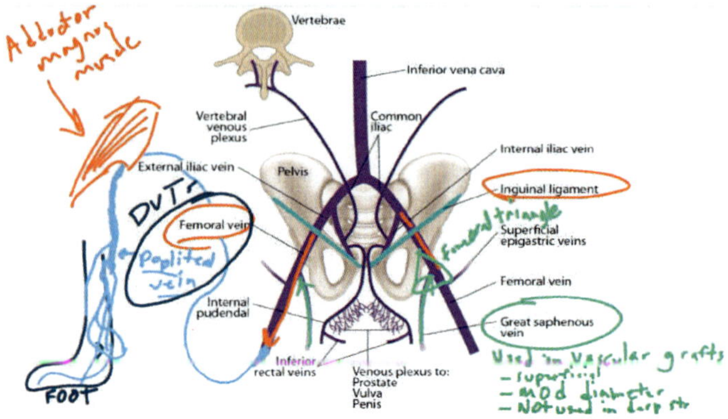

V. Superficial epigastric veins

A. The superficial epigastric veins can form umbilical varices in conjunction with the re-canalized paraumbilical veins.

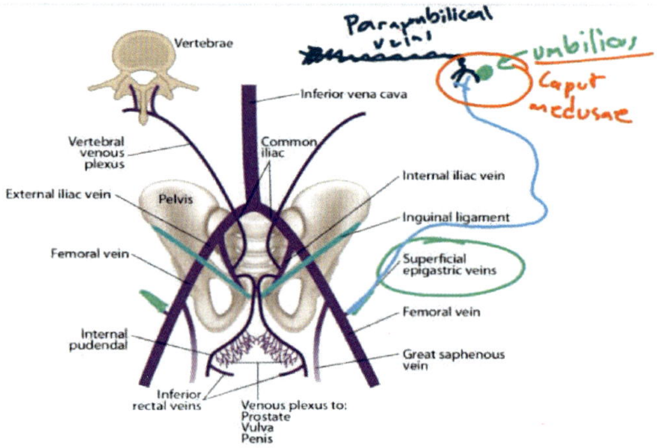

VI. Femoral Triangle

A. Formed by sartorius (lateral), adductor longus (medial), and inguinal ligament (superior)

B. Contains 3 important structures

1. Femoral nerve (most lateral)

2. Femoral artery

3. Femoral vein (most medial)

C. Memory hook: "Swords for naval cadets"

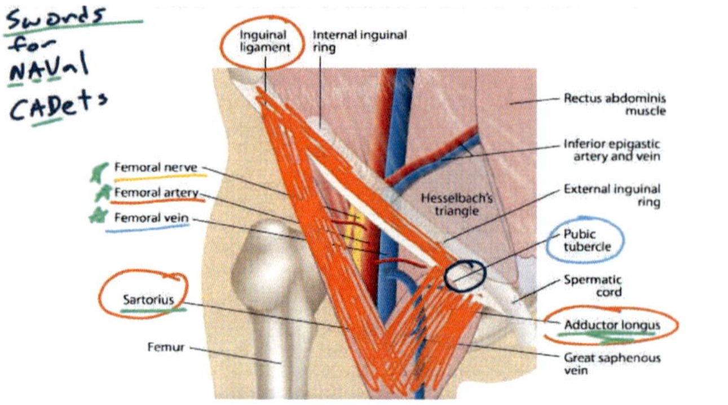

REVIEW QUESTIONS

1. A 45-year-old man with a long history of intermittent and painful hemorrhoids presents to clinic and reports bright red blood per rectum. A rectal exam is performed which confirms the presence of a hemorrhoid. The vein responsible for this eventually drains into which of the following structures?

   A) Great saphenous vein
   B) Femoral vein
   C) External iliac vein
   D) Internal iliac vein

- **Answer: This man has *painful* hemorrhoids, indicating they are external, below the pectinate line. The inferior rectal vein drains the rectum below the pectinate line. The inferior rectal vein drains to the internal pudendal veins, which drain to the internal iliac veins (choice D).**
  - **The great saphenous vein (choice A) drains into the femoral vein (choice B) in the femoral triangle. Neither drain the internal pudendal veins.**
  - **The external iliac veins (choice C) do not receive the internal pudendal veins.**

2. A 65-year-old woman is about to undergo a coronary artery bypass graft (CABG). The surgeon intends to use the great saphenous vein to create the bypass. During the operation, the surgeon identifies the vessel the target vein drains into. What muscle lies medial to this juncture? What major nerve is lateral to this juncture?

- **Answer: The surgeon identified the femoral vein. The great saphenous vein drains into the femoral vein within the femoral triangle. The question is really asking the reader to identify which muscle forms the medial border of the femoral triangle.**
- **Recall the memory hook, "Swords for naval cadets": Sartorius, femoral nerve, artery and vein, and adductor longus.**
- **The next part of the question asks what major nerve lies lateral to this juncture?**
- **That is the femoral nerve, which answers our question.**

Swords for NAVal cADets — Femoral nerve; Adductor longus; Femoral vein

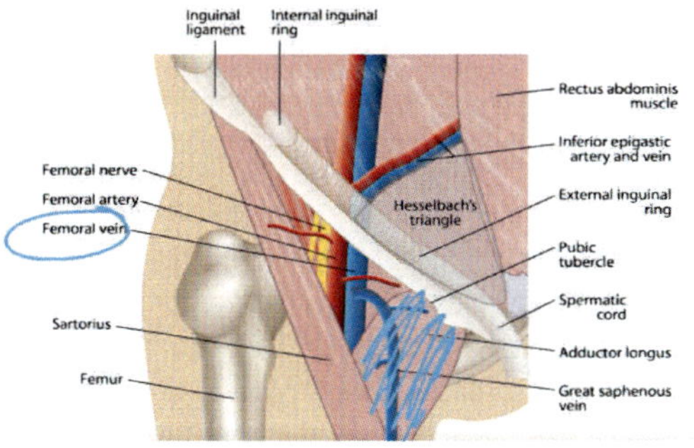

Section V - Gastrointestinal Arteries

I. Foregut, Midgut, and Hindgut

A. Foregut (celiac trunk)

1. Lower esophagus, stomach and first part of duodenum

B. Midgut (SMA)

1. Small intestines, ascending colon, proximal ⅔ of transverse colon

C. Hindgut (IMA)

1. Distal ⅓ of transverse colon, descending and sigmoid colon and rectum

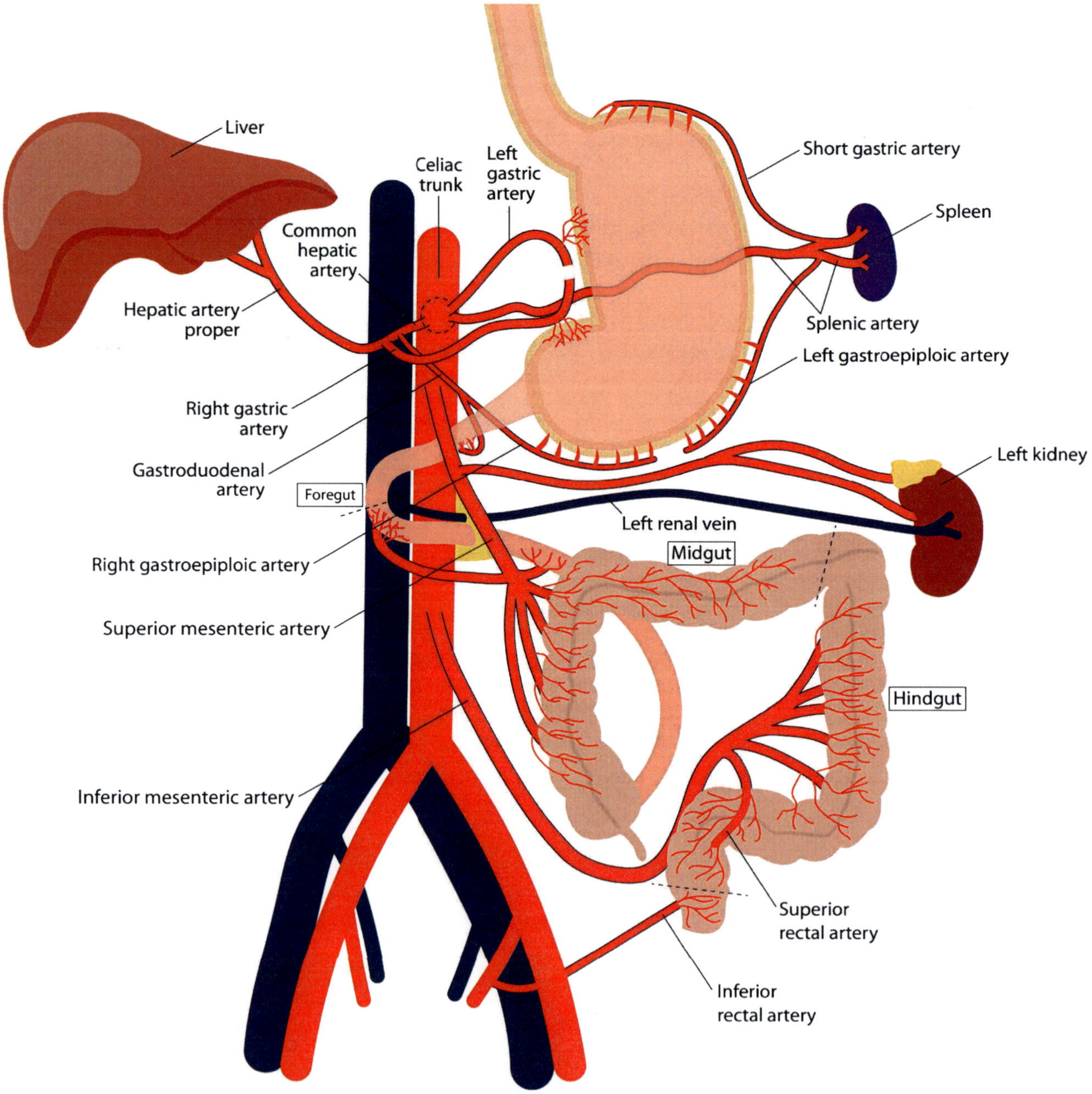

Figure 3.1.8 - Gastrointestinal arteries

Vessel	Anatomy	Notes
Celiac trunk	• Three arteries: left gastric, common hepatic, and, splenic • Supplies foregut, spleen and liver	• Gastroduodenal artery hemorrhage with posterior duodenal ulcers • Hepatic artery proper is part of portal triad • Right + left gastric artery hemorrhage with gastric ulcers • Gastric fundus ischemia with splenic artery obstruction
Superior mesenteric artery (SMA)	• Branches off aorta near the L1 vertebral level • Supplies midgut	• SMA compresses 3rd part of duodenum (SMA syndrome) • 3rd part of duodenum compresses SMA • SMA compresses left renal vein (nutcracker syndrome) • Acute mesenteric ischemia
Inferior mesenteric artery (IMA)	• Supplies hindgut	• Acute mesenteric ischemia (less common than SMA)

Table 3.1.5 - Gastrointestinal arteries

II. Superior Mesenteric Artery (SMA) Syndrome

A. The 3rd part of the duodenum crosses the aorta, causing it to be sandwiched between the superior mesenteric artery and the aorta. There is a fat pad in this region that cushions the duodenum from compression between these two arterial structures. With loss of cushioning fat, the duodenum can be compressed, leading to a small bowel obstruction (SBO).

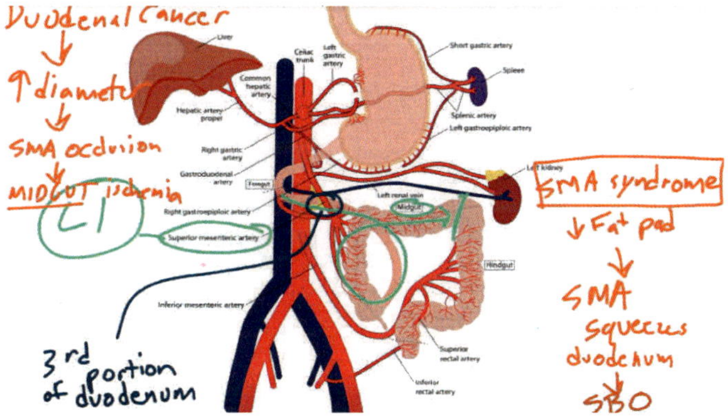

REVIEW QUESTIONS ?

1. A 47-year-old male presents with worsening upper abdominal pain. Endoscopy of the stomach is performed and reveals an ulcer in an area where gastric ulcers are most likely to present. If this ulcer were to perforate, what arterial vessel is susceptible to injury?

Gastric ulcer on lesser curvature (R + L gastric arteries)

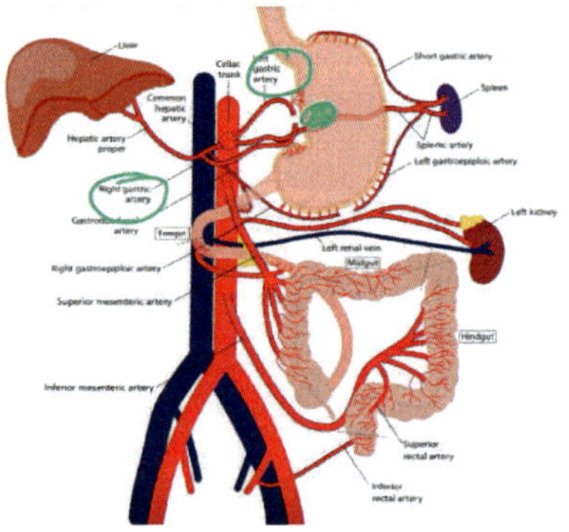

- **Answer: The gastric ulcer in the location where ulcers "are most likely to present", indicating the lesser curvature. The right and left gastric arteries provide blood to the lesser curvature. In the case of ulcer perforation, these vessels are susceptible to hemorrhage.**
  - **Note: If we were talking about a duodenal ulcer on the POSTERIOR duodenum, you should be thinking about hemorrhage of the gastroduodenal artery**

2. A 64-year-old female presents with excruciating abdominal pain. Thorough evaluation reveals complete compression of the duodenum as it crosses the abdominal aorta. Which statement may be true regarding the pathological process?

   A) There is increased fat storage surrounding the area of compression
   B) Arteries supplying the hindgut are responsible for the compressed structure
   C) Compression results in decreased venous drainage of the left kidney
   D) Atherosclerosis is the cause of the intestinal obstruction

- **Answer: The 3rd part of the duodenum is compressed between the aorta and the SMA. An additional structure that crosses here is the left renal vein (choice C).**
- **Choice A is wrong, because fat would be decreased, not increased.**
- **Choice B is wrong because the SMA supplies midgut structures, not hindgut structures.**
- **Choice D is wrong because atherosclerosis is not the root cause of the pathogenesis of this condition.**

Section VI - Gastrointestinal Veins and the Portal System

I. The venous supply of the gastrointestinal system should be conceptually divided into the inferior mesenteric vein, the splenic vein, and the portal vein. (See Table 3.1.6 - Gastrointestinal veins and the portal system)

Vessel	Anatomy	Notes
Inferior mesenteric vein (IMV)	• Drains descending colon and superior rectal veins into splenic vein	• Internal and painless hemorrhoids • Anorectal varices in cirrhosis (anastomosis with inferior rectal veins)
Splenic vein	• Drains spleen and gastric fundus	• Thrombosis → ↑ venous pressure → varices in gastric fundus
Portal vein	• Drains SMV, IMV and splenic vein • Empties into liver	• Hepatic cirrhosis → ↑ portal pressure → ↑ pressure in veins that drain to portal system → varices • Splenic vein: varices of gastric fundus • Left gastric: esophageal varices • Superior rectal vein: anorectal varices • Paraumbilical vein: caput medusae

Table 3.1.6 - Gastrointestinal veins and the portal system

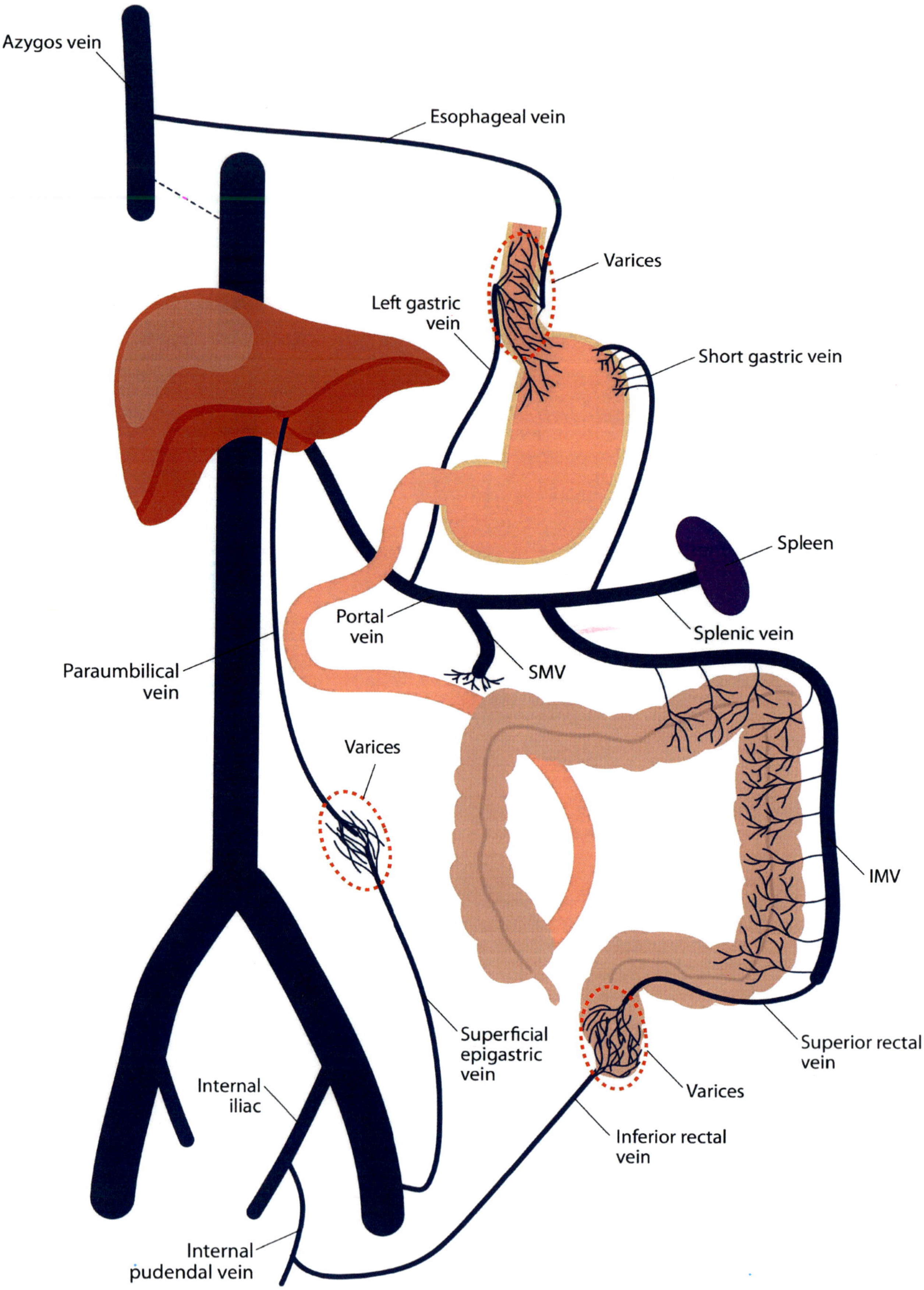

Figure 3.1.9 - Gastrointestinal veins and the portal system

II. Varices of the Gastric Fundus

A. Increased pressure, compression, or thrombosis of the splenic vein can lead to varices in the gastric fundus.

B. These can present similar to esophageal varices. For example, a cirrhotic patient with hematemesis is likely to have esophageal varices. However, they could have varices in the gastric fundus, which makes it a possible distractor for examination purposes.

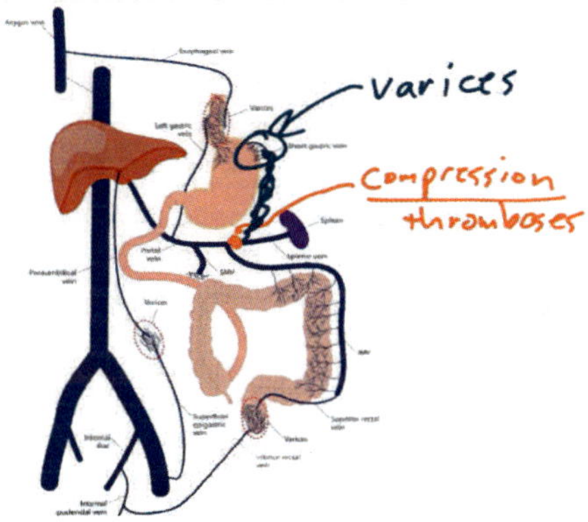

REVIEW QUESTIONS

1. A 55-year-old female with known liver cirrhosis presents with massive hematemesis. Evaluation confirms the presence of ruptured varices. What vein of the portal system is directly involved in the varices? Does it drain into the splenic vein, the portal vein, or the superior mesenteric vein?

Azygos
IVC
Esophageal vein
Anastomosis
Left gastric vein
Portal vein

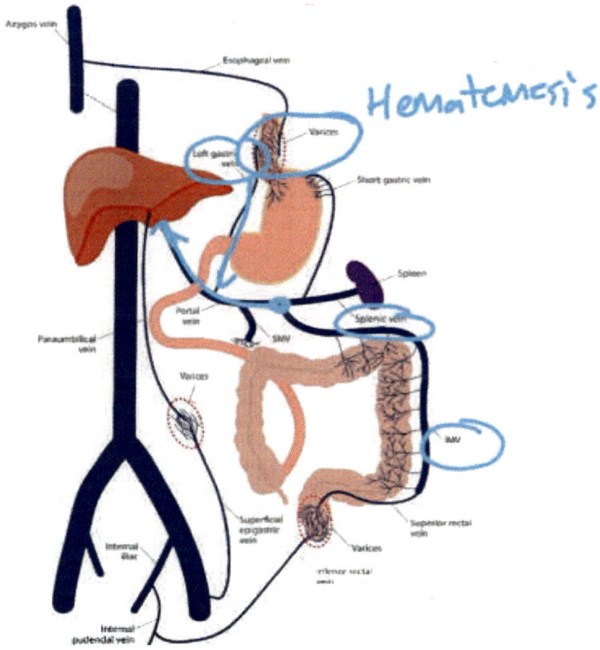

- **Answer: The left gastric vein forms an anastomosis with the esophageal vein, which drains into the azygos vein. The left gastric vein is the vein involved in these varices and drains *directly* into the portal vein.**
- **The splenic vein and the superior mesenteric vein join to form the portal vein. This joining occurs before the left gastric vein drains into the portal network.**

Section VII - Ovarian and Testicular Vasculature

I. The vascular supply to the gonads is straight forward in terms of naming. Consider the ovarian artery and vein as well as the testicular artery and vein. (See Table 3.1.7 - Ovarian and testicular vasculature)

Vessel	Anatomy	Notes
Ovarian artery	• Ovarian arteries both branch from aorta	• Ovarian torsion blocks ovarian artery
Ovarian vein	• Veins drain ovaries (right to IVC; left to left renal vein)	• Vein thrombosis in septic pelvic thrombophlebitis
Testicular vein	• Pampiniform plexus → testicular veins (right to IVC; left to left renal vein)	• Decreased drainage → varicocele • Left renal cancer can cause left varicocele
Testicular artery	• Branch from aorta • Supplies testes	• Testicular torsion blocks testicular artery

Table 3.1.7 - Ovarian and testicular vasculature

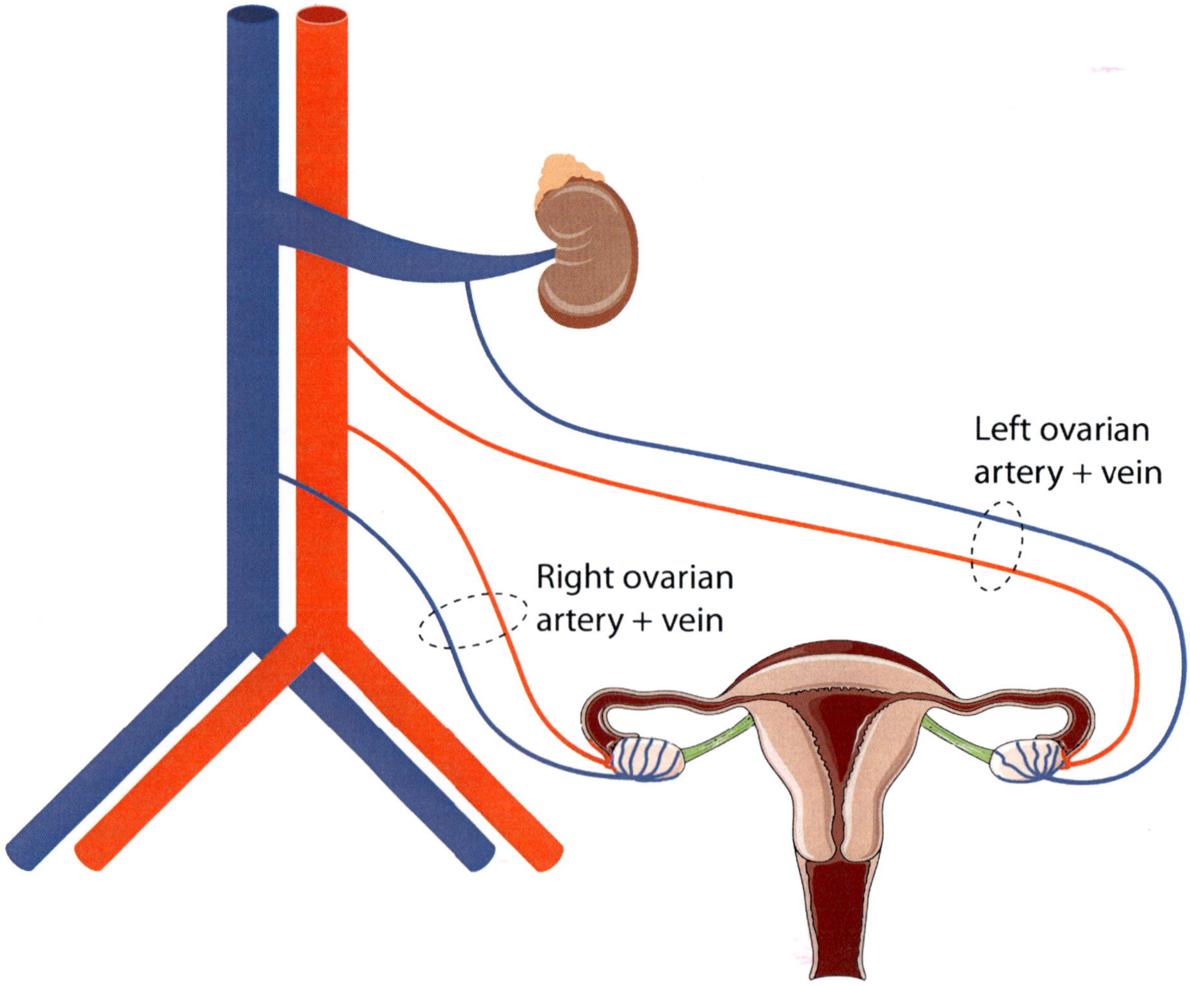

Figure 3.1.10 - Ovarian vasculature

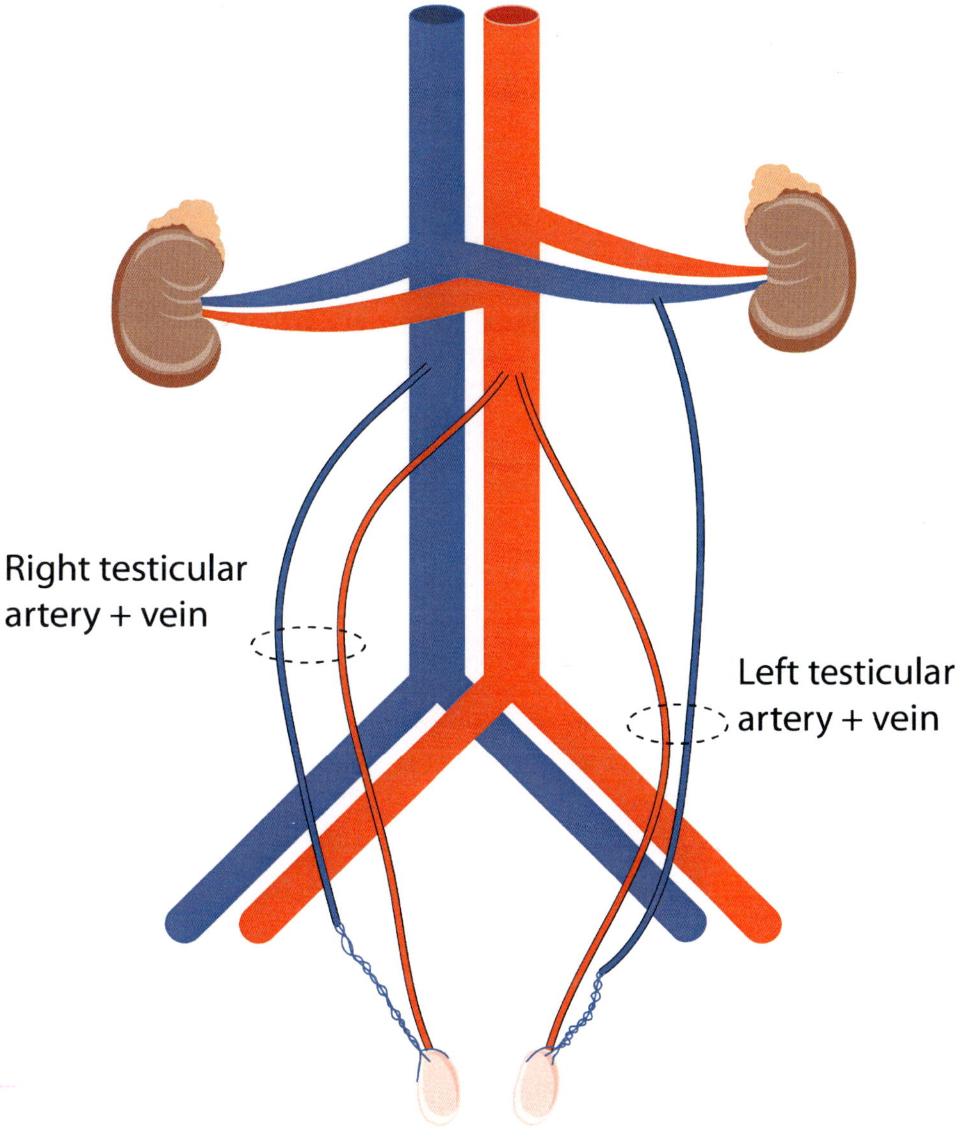

Figure 3.1.11 - Testicular vasculature

II. Septic Pelvic Thrombophlebitis (SPT)

A. Occurs in postpartum women. Pregnant patients are at higher risk for clotting and developing these thromboses. These thromboses form in pelvic veins, especially in the ovarian veins and become a nidus for infection (sepsis).

B. This is very rare. Endometritis, infection of the uterus, is much more likely to cause sepsis in a postpartum patient. However, SPT can be a clever distractor on board exams.

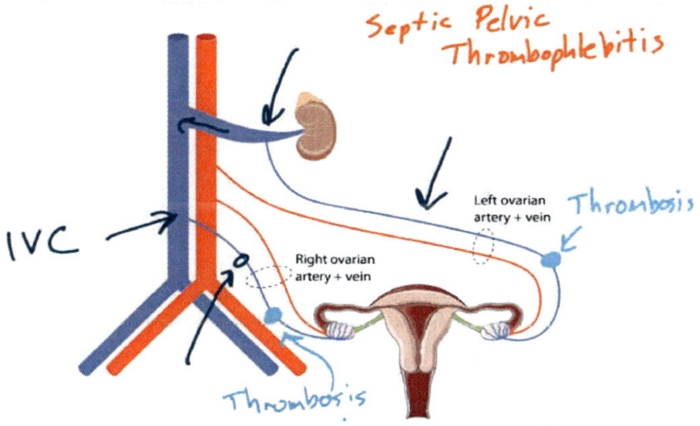

REVIEW QUESTIONS

1. A 22-year-old male presents with excruciating right testicular pain. Physical exam demonstrates that the testicle has wrapped around the spermatic cord. Doppler ultrasound reveals decreased blood flow through the testicular artery and the presence of venous congestion. What vascular path would this deoxygenated blood normally follow to reach the heart?

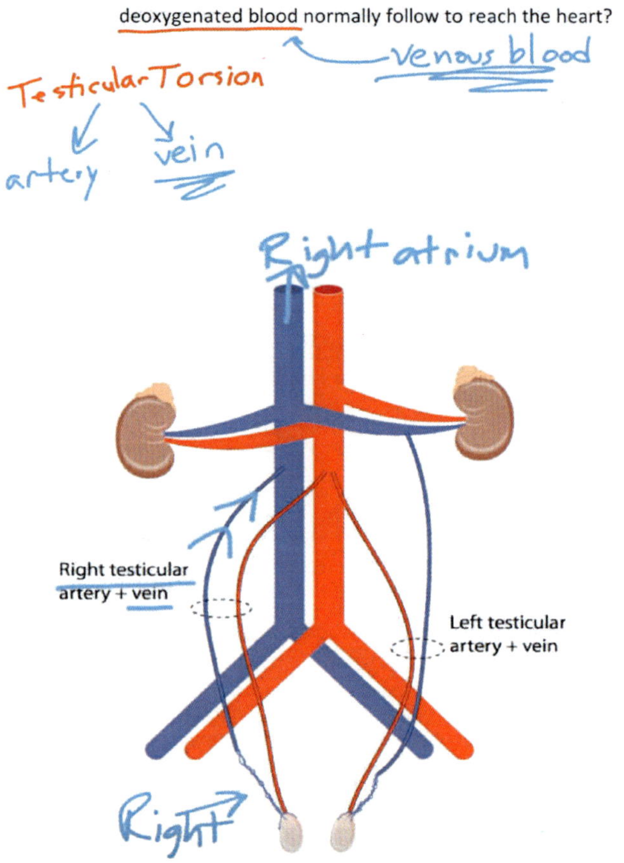

- **Answer: This patient has testicular torsion, a condition in which the testicular artery is compressed and the testicle is ischemic. In addition to testicular arteries, the testicular vein can also be compressed. The question stem states, "deoxygenated blood" which indicates the blood has already been delivered to the tissues, venous blood. Blood drained by the *right* testicular vein goes directly to the IVC before being taken up to the right atrium.**
  - **Note: The left testicular vein drains to the left renal vein before reaching the IVC.**

Section VIII - Cardiovascular Anatomy on Imaging

I. Recognizing cardiovascular structures on imaging can be difficult. The best way to become good at recognition is through practice questions. This section utilizes a strictly question-based method to assist in acquiring this skill.

REVIEW QUESTIONS

1. A 63-year-old male with possible renal calculus undergoes an abdominal CT scan. The radiologist confirms the presence of renal calculi and identifies the region with an arrow. This patient has a history of a pulmonary embolism following a deep vein thrombosis. Through which structure did the embolism travel to the lungs?

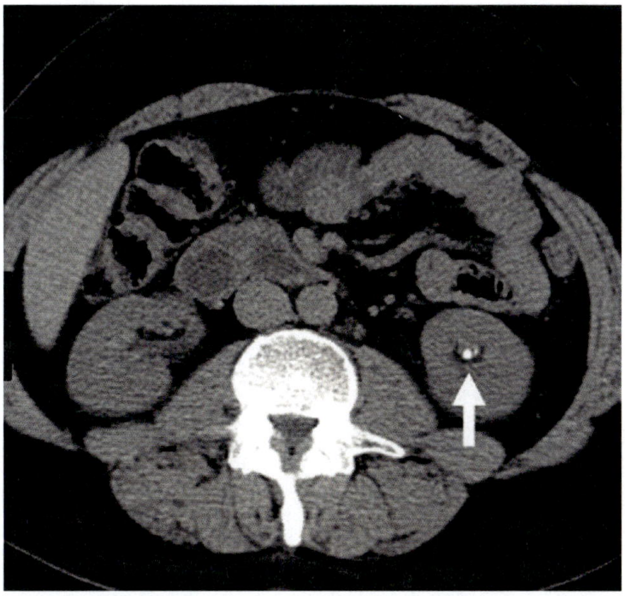

By Kristie Guite, Louis Hinshaw and Fred Lee [CC BY 3.0 (https://creativecommons.org/licenses/by/3.0)], via Wikimedia Commons

- **Answer: The arrow indicates the calculus in the kidney. The patient had a deep vein thrombosis (DVT) which embolized to the lungs. Deep vein thromboemboli will travel through the inferior vena cava before ultimately reaching the lungs. So, which structure in this image demonstrates the IVC? The structure indicated by the blue circle. Remember that the IVC will *ascend* on the right. And the aorta (red circle) will *descend* on the left.**

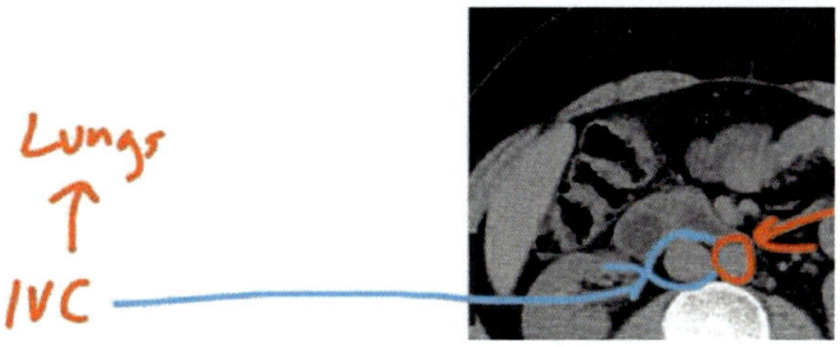

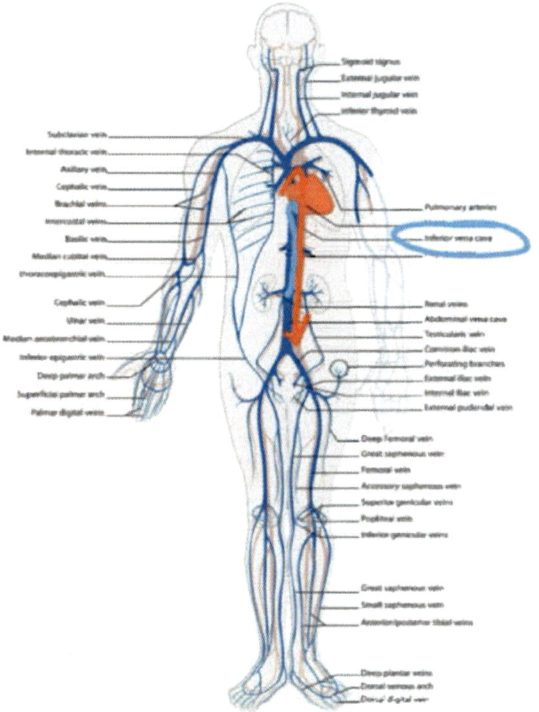

By LadyofHats, Mariana Ruiz Villarreal [Public domain], via Wikimedia Commons

REVIEW QUESTIONS

2. A patient experiences a massive pulmonary embolism, indicated in the image with red arrows. Identify the major vessel which carries deoxygenated blood to the right atrium.

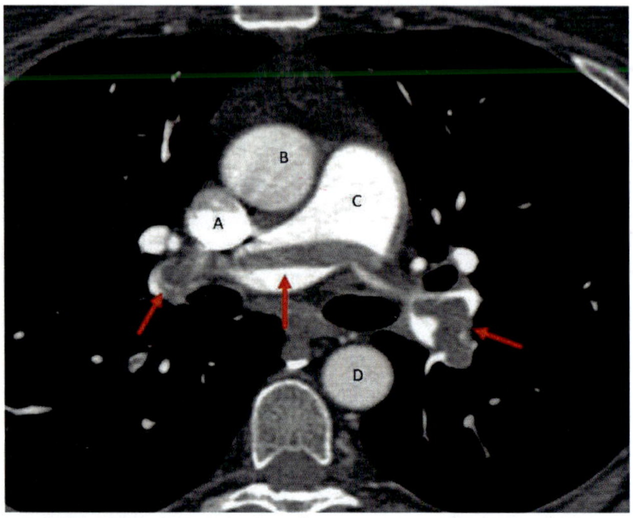

By Carlcl at fr.wikipedia [CC BY-SA 2.5 (https://creativecommons.org/licenses/by-sa/2.5)], from Wikimedia Commons

- **Answer: The location of the pulmonary embolus is already labeled. The question is really asking: Which of the following of these 4 structures carries deoxygenated blood to the right atrium?**

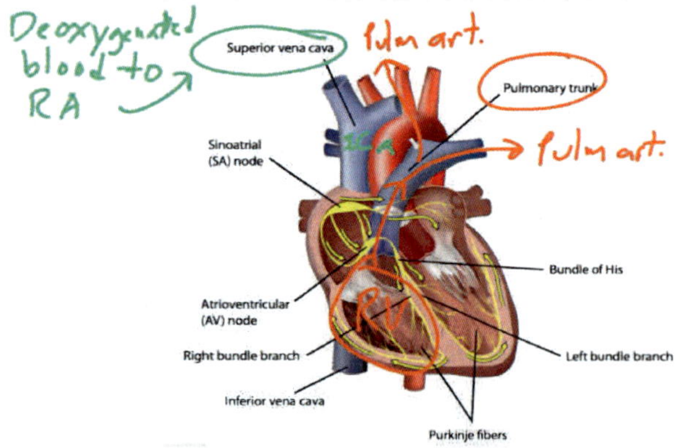

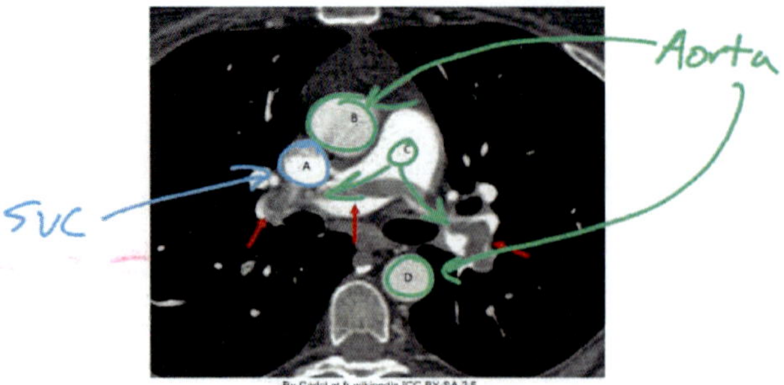

By Carlcl at fr.wikipedia [CC BY-SA 2.5 (https://creativecommons.org/licenses/by-sa/2.5)], from Wikimedia Commons

- **Blood leaves the right ventricle, enter the pulmonary trunk, and then split into both the left pulmonary artery and the left pulmonary artery. The superior vena cava (SVC) will carry deoxygenated blood from the upper part of the body and deliver it to the right atrium.**
- **Choice B (ascending aorta) and choice D (descending aorta) will carry *oxygenated* blood away from the heart.**
- **Choice C will carry deoxygenated blood *away* from the right ventricle.**
- **Choice A, the SVC, is the only structure that carries *deoxygenated* blood *to* the right atrium. So the answer is A, the SVC**

REVIEW QUESTIONS

3. A man presents with duodenal obstruction secondary to compression between two major blood vessels. Identify these two structures. Besides the duodenum, what other structure can be compressed by these two structures?

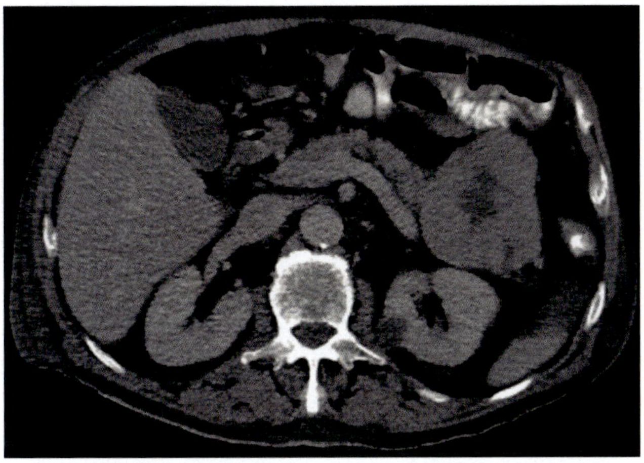

By James Heilman, MD [CC BY-SA 3.0 (https://creativecommons.org/licenses/by-sa/3.0)], from Wikimedia Commons

- **Answer: This man has duodenal obstruction due to compression between the SMA and the abdominal aorta.**

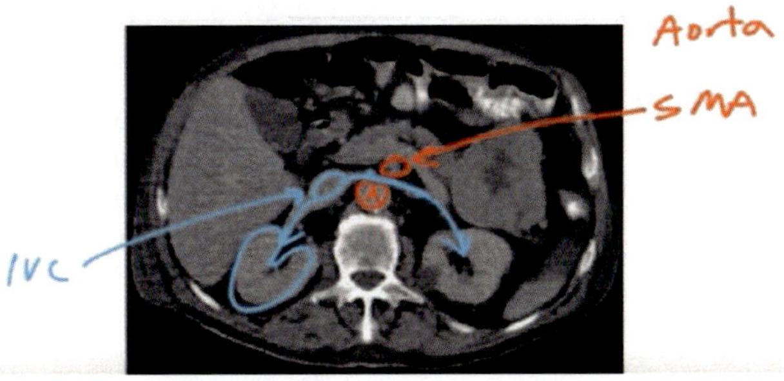

- **The aorta is indicated by the circle with an "A" inside it.**
- **The SMA is indicated by the small circle.**
- **The IVC is indicated by the blue circle.**
- **Therefore, we have found both structures causing the compression. In addition to the 3rd portion of the duodenum, the left renal vein (blue line between both red circles) can be compressed.**

4. A 23-year-old male with an upper respiratory infection obtains a chest x-ray. The physician shows the patient the radiograph and proceeds to answer questions regarding what is shown. Identify the aortic arch, the right atrium and the right ventricle.

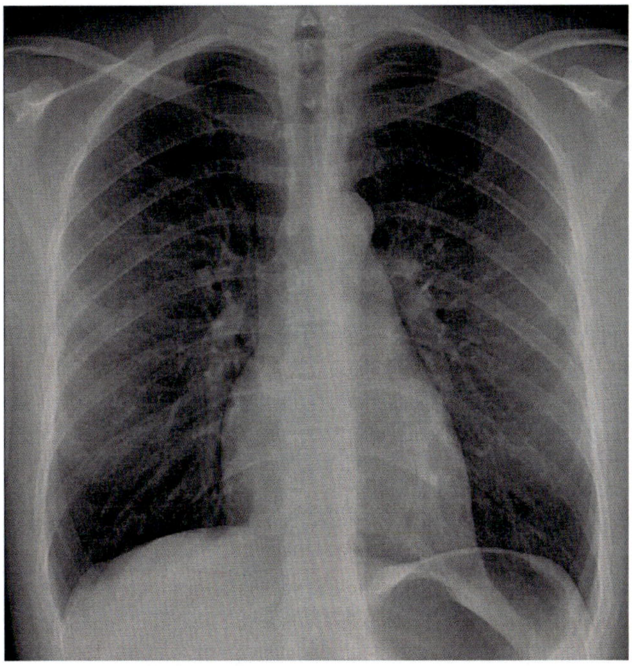

By Mikael Häggström [CC0], from Wikimedia Commons

- **Answer: On chest x-rays, identify the aortic arch as the notch at the top left of the cardiac silhouette. Identify the right atrium as the upper bump on the patient's right. And identify the right ventricle as the lower bump on the patient's right.**

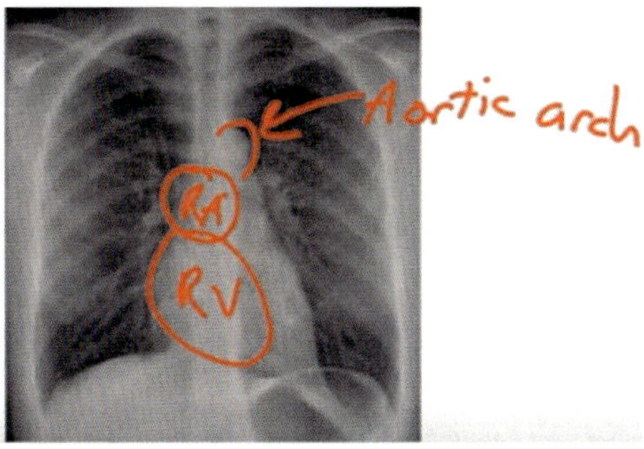

RESPIRATORY ANATOMY

Section I - Overview of Respiratory Anatomy

I. Basic Principles

A. Anatomy

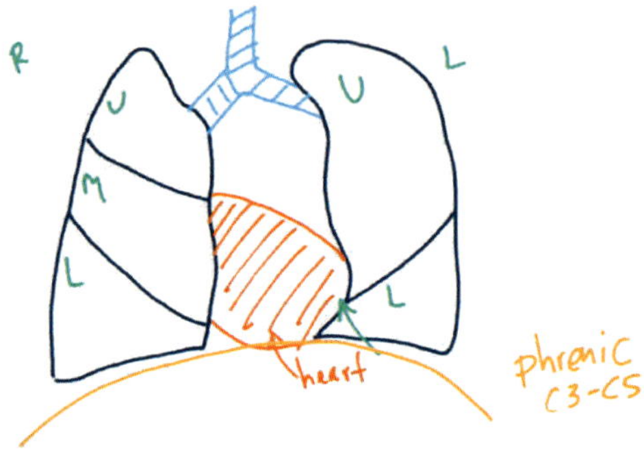

1. Lobe locations
   a) Right lung (three lobes)
   b) Left lung (two lobes)
2. Diaphragm
   a) Innervated by the phrenic nerve
3. Respiratory tree
   a) Gross anatomy and histology (see Figures 3.1 and 3.2)
4. Conducting zone
   a) The mucociliary escalator is comprised of the pseudostratified ciliated columnar epithelium and mucus from the goblet cells, and is important in clearing debris.
   b) Goblet cells
      (1) Located in the trachea, bronchi, and bronchioles
      (2) Produce mucus
   c) Club cells
5. Respiratory zone
   a) Type I pneumocytes

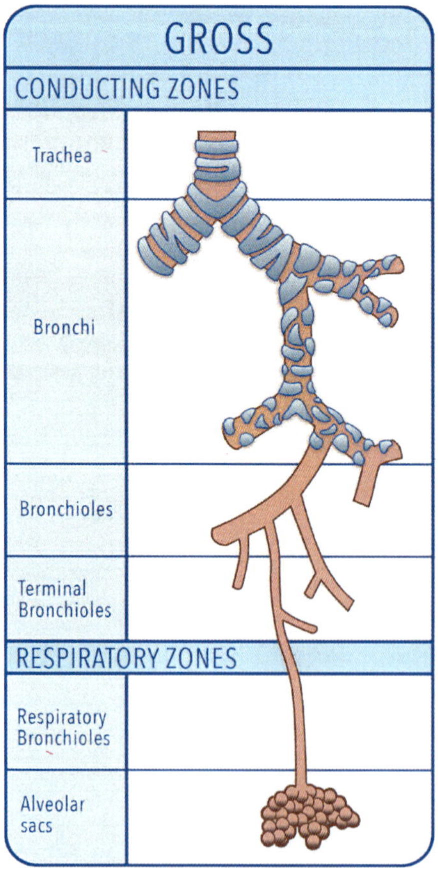

Figure 3.2.1 - Anatomy of the respiratory tree

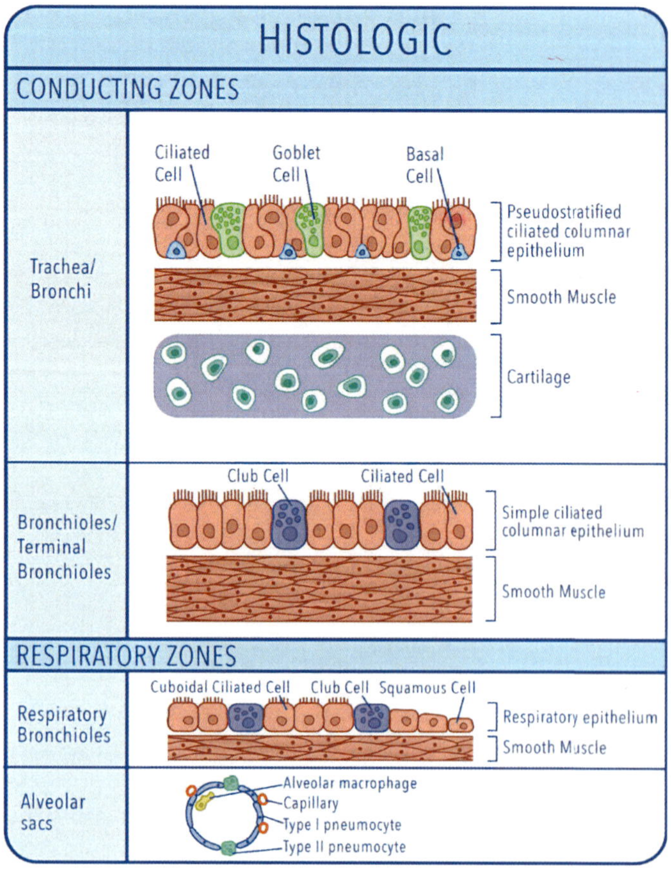

Figure 3.2.2 - Histology of the respiratory tree

b) Type II pneumocytes

    (1) Produce surfactant which contains the lipid called dipalmitoylphosphatidylcholine (DPPC)

    (2) Proliferate when the lungs are damaged

c) Alveolar macrophages

REVIEW QUESTIONS ?

1. What nerve innervates the diaphragm?

    - **The phrenic nerve (C3-C5)**

2. An x-ray reveals an elevation of the left hemidiaphragm. Is the left or right phrenic nerve damaged?

    - **The phrenic nerve is responsible for allowing the diaphragm to contract downwards**
    - **Elevation of the left hemidiaphragm can indicate damage to the L phrenic nerve**

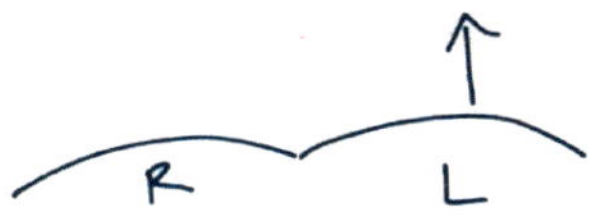

3. Why are patients who take TNF-alpha inhibitors at an increased risk of mycobacterium tuberculosis?

    - **TNF-alpha is released from macrophages and assists in granuloma formation.**
    - **TNF-alpha inhibitors → breakdown of granuloma → ↑ risk of TB**

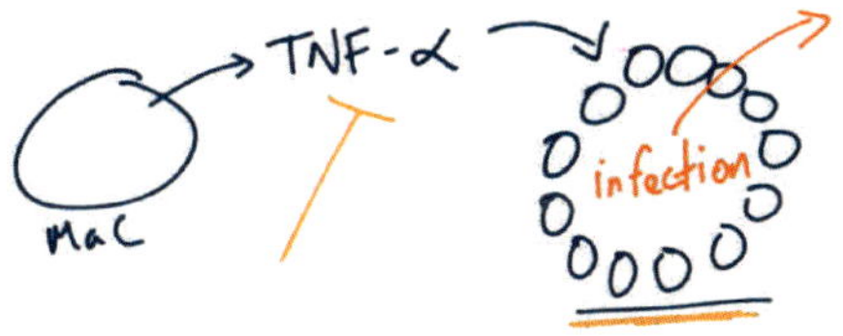

4. What genetic disorder results in destruction of the alveolar walls?

    - **Alpha-1 antitrypsin deficiency → ↑ elastase activity → emphysema**

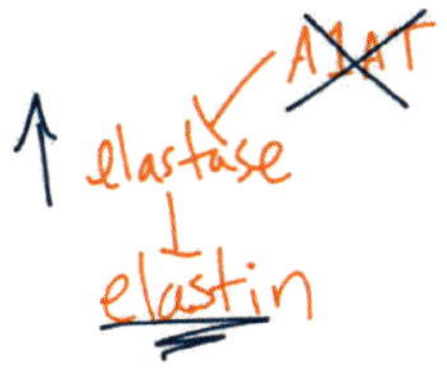

REVIEW QUESTIONS

5. What histological changes would occur in the conducting zone as a result of chronic bronchitis?

- **Chronic bronchitis → chronic irritation → metaplasia**
- **Pseudostratified ciliated columnar epithelium → stratified squamous epithelium**
- **Goblet cells → hypertrophy → ↑ mucus**

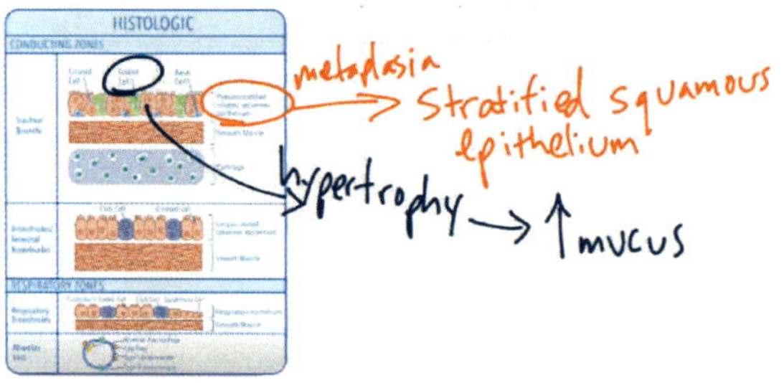

6. What disease is a result of a defective dynein arm?

- **Kartagener syndrome**

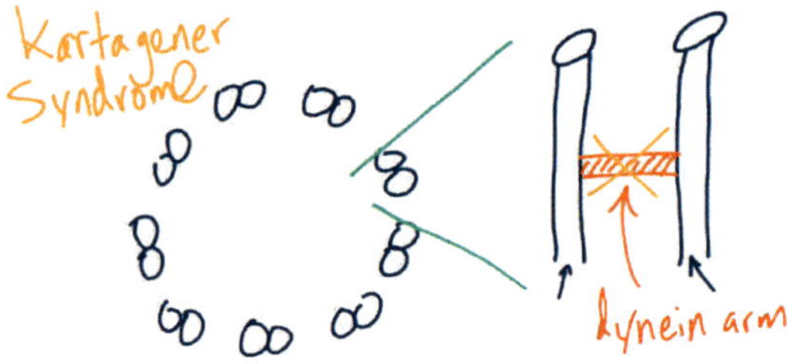

7. How can the lecithin to sphingomyelin ratio be used to determine the maturity of fetal lungs?

- **Lecithin and sphingomyelin are components of surfactant (necessary for optimal lung function)**
- **Lecithin steadily rises throughout pregnancy while sphingomyelin stays relatively constant → ↑ L:S ratio**
- **L:S > 2 → mature lungs**
- **L:S < 1.5 → immature lungs**

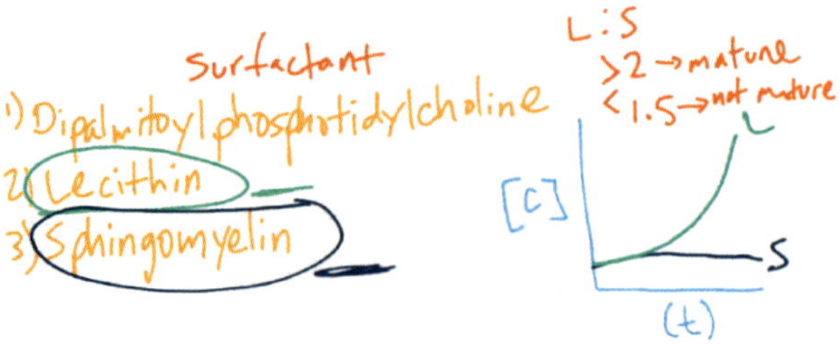

8. What substances increase/decrease the synthesis of surfactant?

- **Steroids ↑ surfactant**
- **Insulin ↓ surfactant**

cortisol → ↑ surfactant
insulin → ↓ surfactant NRDS
maternal diabetes → fetal hyperglycemia → ↑ insulin → ↓ surfactant

9. How would maternal diabetes would impact the development of the infant's lungs?

- **Insulin decreases surfactant production.**
- **Maternal diabetes → maternal and fetal hyperglycemia → ↑ fetal insulin production → ↓ fetal surfactant → ↓ lung development**

10. What cells would be involved in attempting to remove asbestos bodies?

- **Particles larger than 2 micrometers are removed by the mucociliary escalator**
- **Particles smaller than 2 micrometers are removed by alveolar macrophages**
- **Asbestos bodies are small → removed by alveolar macrophages**

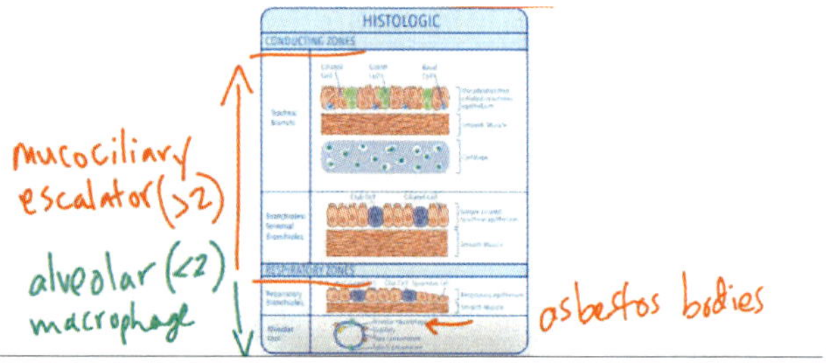

RENAL ANATOMY

Section I - Overview of Renal Anatomy

I. Basic Principles

A. Primary functions of the kidneys

1. Removal of waste products (drugs, urea, etc.)
2. Electrolyte homeostasis
3. Acid-base regulation
4. Blood volume homeostasis
5. Regulation of erythropoiesis
6. Regulation of blood pressure
7. Regulation of bone health (vitamin D, calcium, and phosphorous)

B. Anatomy

1. Figure 3.3.1 provides a basic overview of the anatomy of the kidney.

a) The functional unit of the kidney is the nephron (Figure 3.3.2), which consists of several important segments.

(1) Proximal convoluted tubule (PCT)

(2) Thin descending limb of the loop of Henle

(3) Thin ascending limb of the loop of Henle

(4) Thick ascending limb of the loop of Henle (TAL)

(5) Distal convoluted tubule (DCT)

(6) Collecting duct

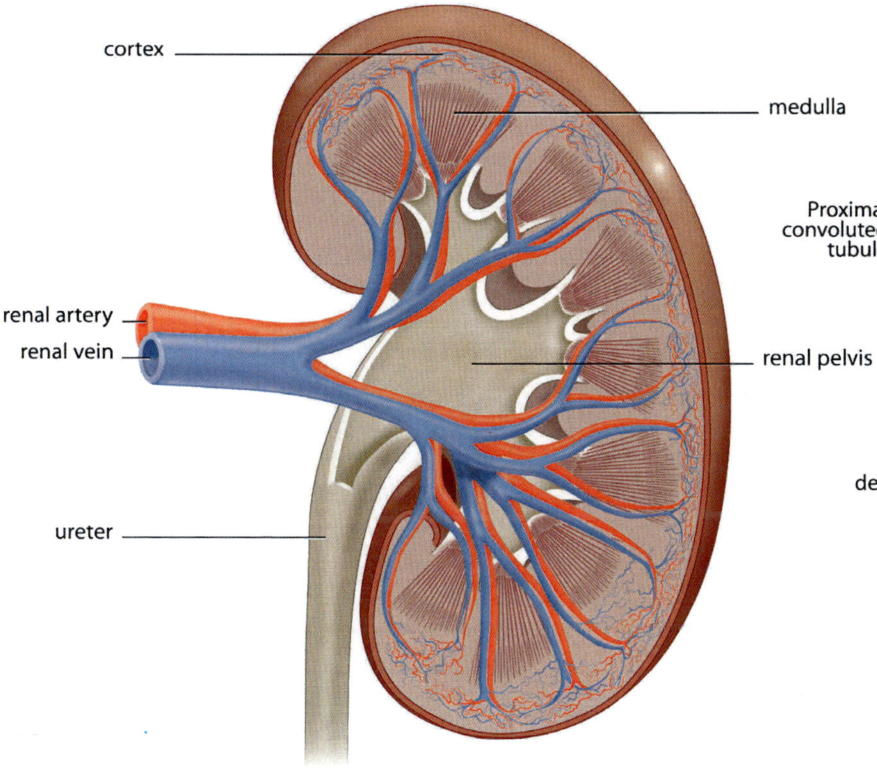

Figure 3.3.1 - Anatomy of the kidney

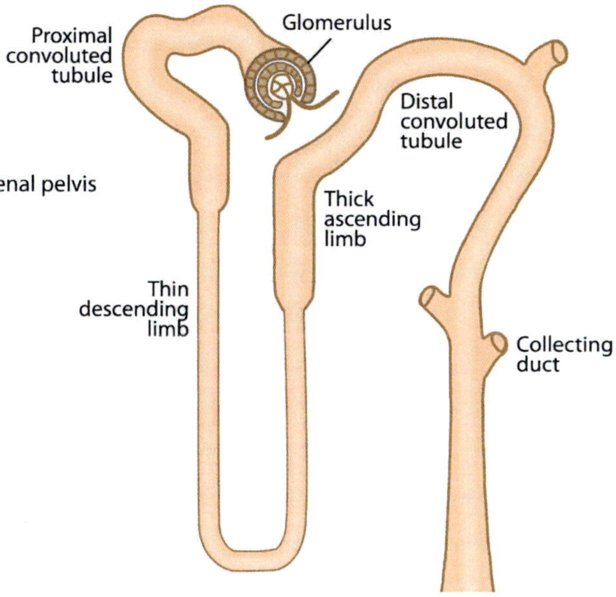

Figure 3.3.2 - Anatomy of the nephron

2. The first portion of the nephron is the glomerulus (Figures 3.3.3 & 3.3.4).
   a) The afferent arteriole contains blood that enters the glomerulus, and the efferent arteriole contains blood that leaves the glomerulus.
   b) The glomerular basement membrane is composed of negatively charged glycoproteins, which prevent filtration of like-charged proteins.
   c) The podocytes contain fenestrations that are small in diameter and prevent filtration of large molecules. The podocytes are also negatively charged, which prevent filtration of like-charged molecules.

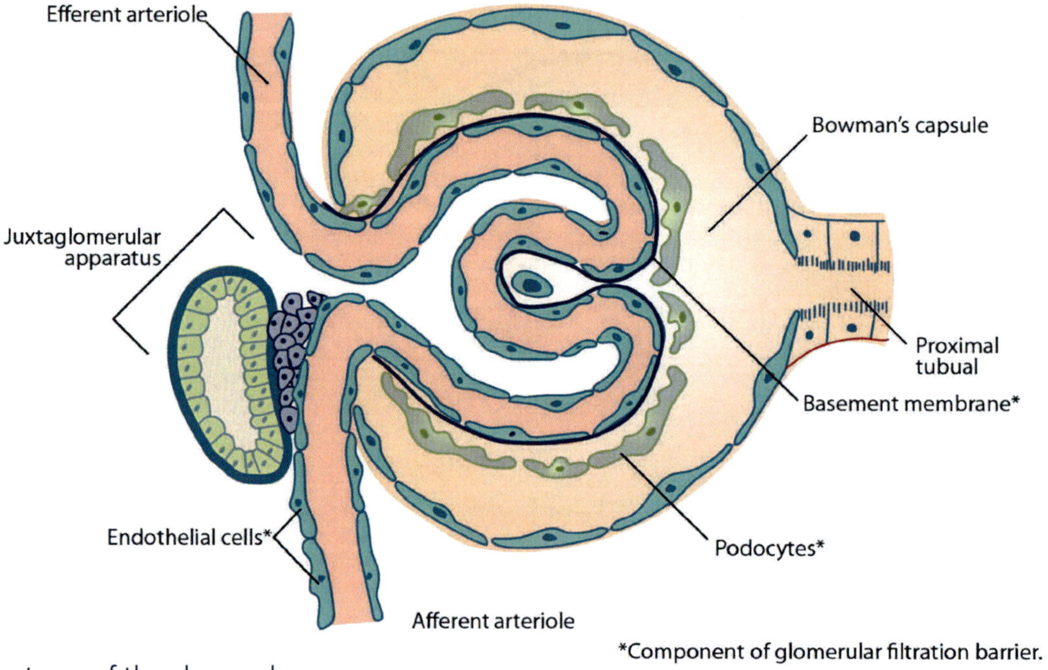

Figure 3.3.3 - Anatomy of the glomerulus

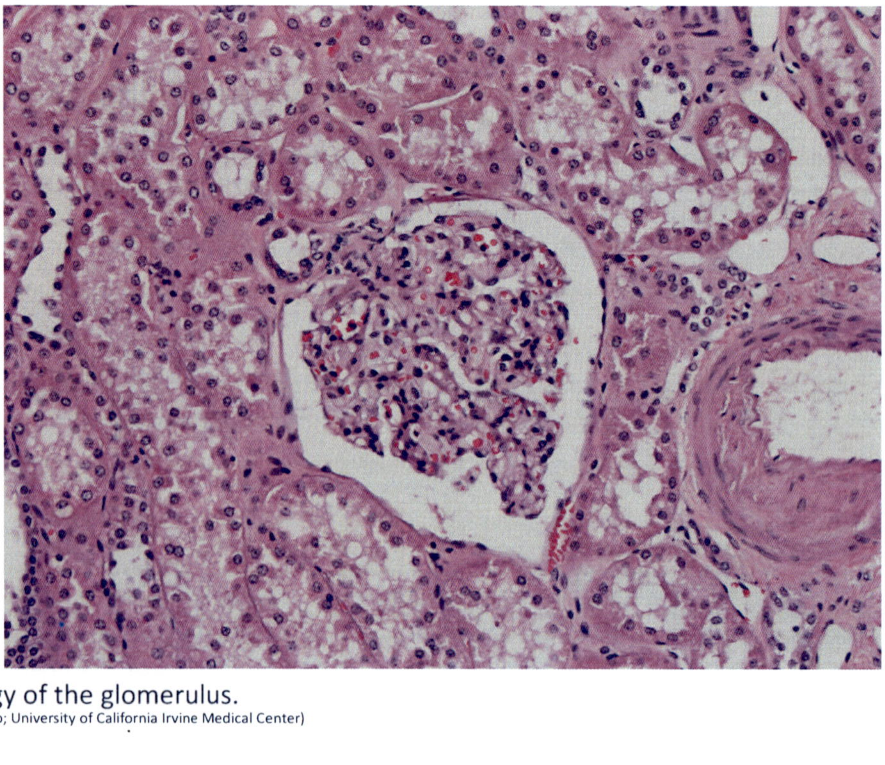

Figure 3.3.4 - Histology of the glomerulus.
(Courtesy of Roberto Alvaro A. Taguibao; University of California Irvine Medical Center)

REVIEW QUESTIONS

1. Which gender has a shorter urethra and how is this clinically relevant?

   - **Answer: Females have shorter urethras, making ascending infections to the bladder more likely.**
     - **Note: Ureters have angles and valves to prevent bladder infections to ascend up to the kidneys. Abnormalities of the ureters can permit bladder infection (cystitis) to reach the kidneys (pyelonephritis).**

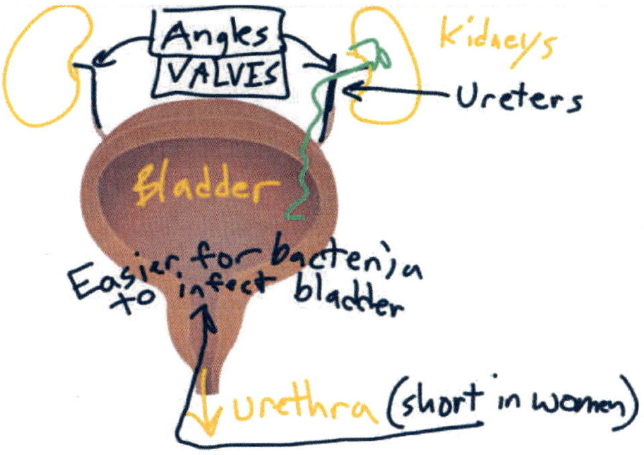

GASTROINTESTINAL ANATOMY

Section I - Mesentery and Peritoneum

I. Peritoneum

A. Visceral peritoneum lines the organs

B. Parietal peritoneum lines the rest of the cavity

C. Sagittal View of the Mesentery and Peritoneum

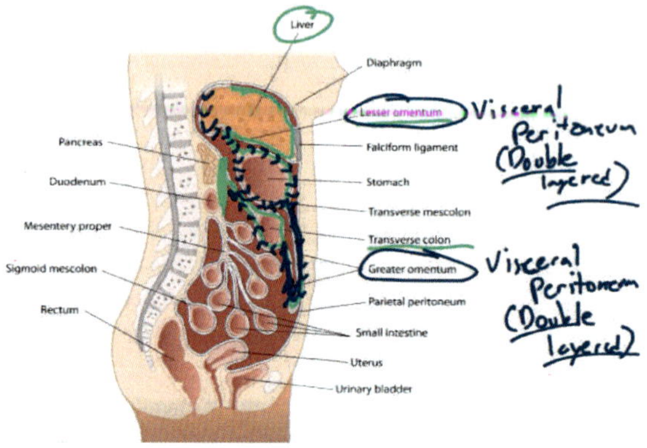

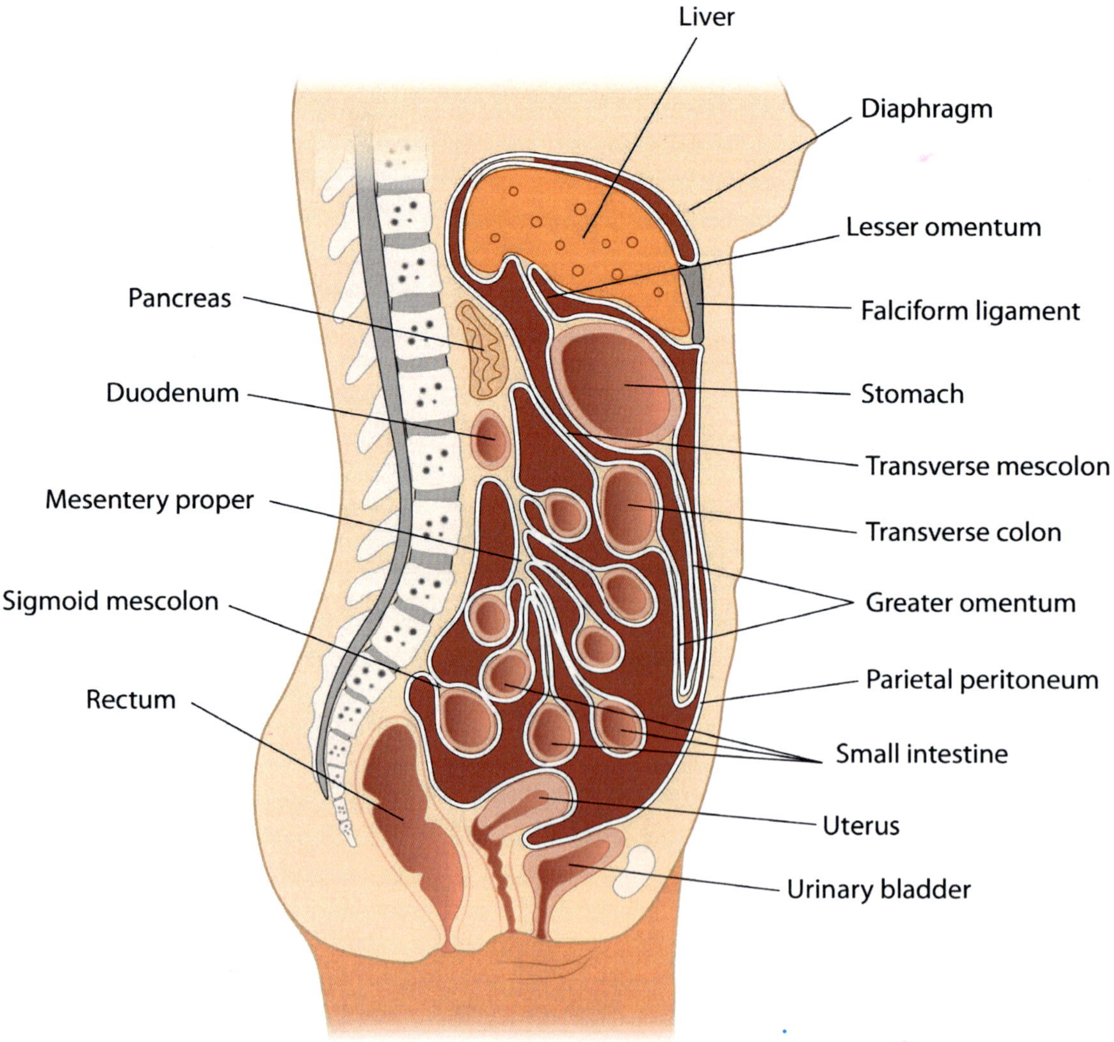

Figure 3.4.1 - Sagittal View of the Mesentery and Peritoneum

II. Mesentery

A. Double layer of peritoneum

B. Contains arteries and veins that supply intestinal tract

C. Examples:

1. Lesser omentum
2. Greater omentum

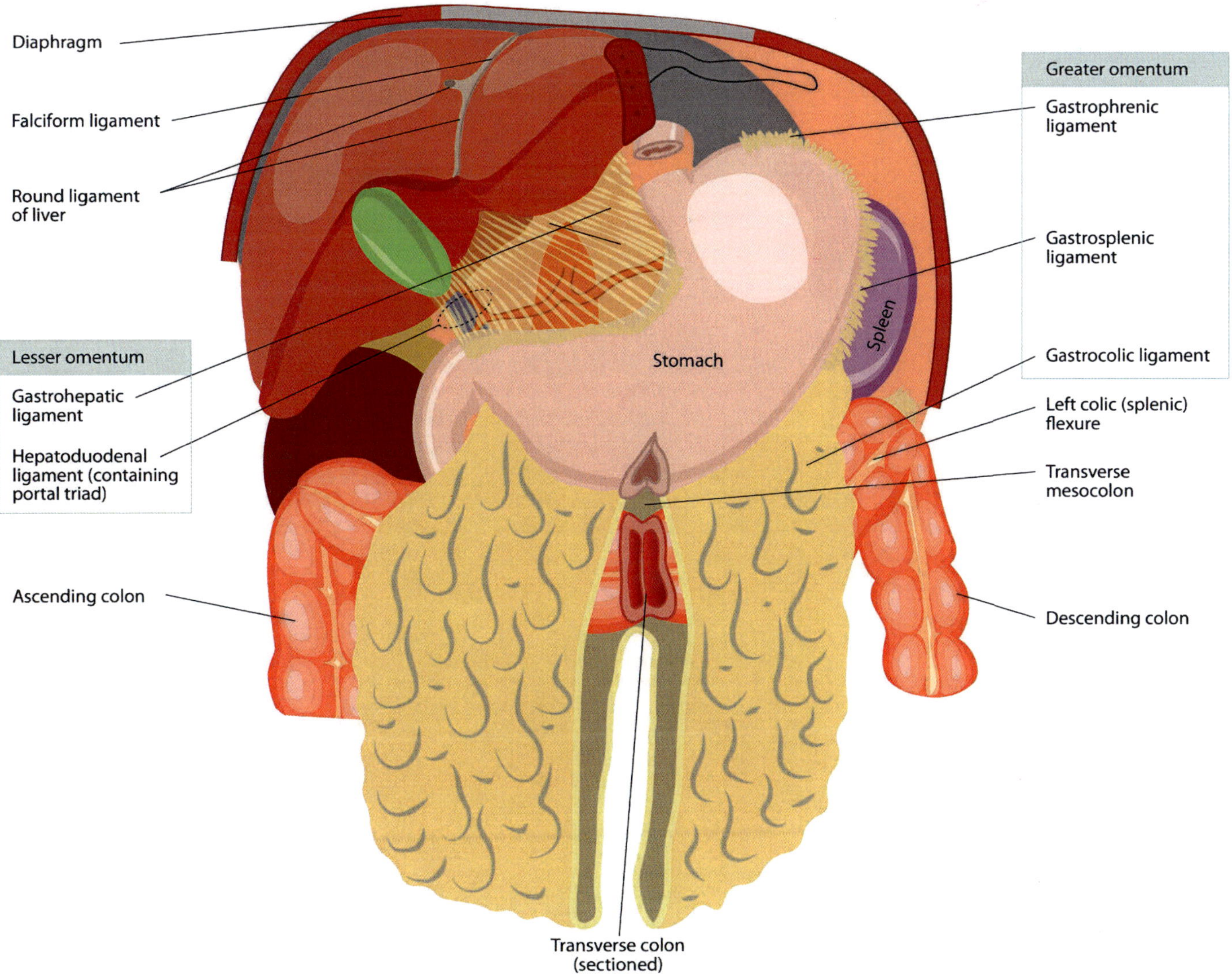

Figure 3.4.2 - Anterior view of the mesentery

Structure	Location	Notes
Lesser omentum (hepatogastric ligament)	• From liver to lesser curvature of stomach	• Contains gastric vessels
Lesser omentum (hepatoduodenal ligament)	• From liver to proximal duodenum	• Pringle maneuver (temporary clamp portal triad to reduce bleeding from liver) • Contains portal triad (hepatic artery proper, portal vein and common bile duct)
Greater omentum (gastrocolic ligament)	• From greater curvature of stomach to transverse colon	• The ascending and descending colon are retroperitoneal → doesn't connect to greater omentum
Greater omentum (gastrosplenic ligament)	• From greater curvature of stomach to spleen	• Contains branches of splenic artery and vein (short gastrics and left gastro-omental)
Splenorenal ligament	• From spleen to posterior abdominal wall	• Contains splenic artery and vein
Falciform ligament	• From anterior liver to abdominal wall	• Contains paraumbilical veins (forms caput medusae with superficial epigastric veins)

Table 3.4.1 - Peritoneal and mesenteric structures

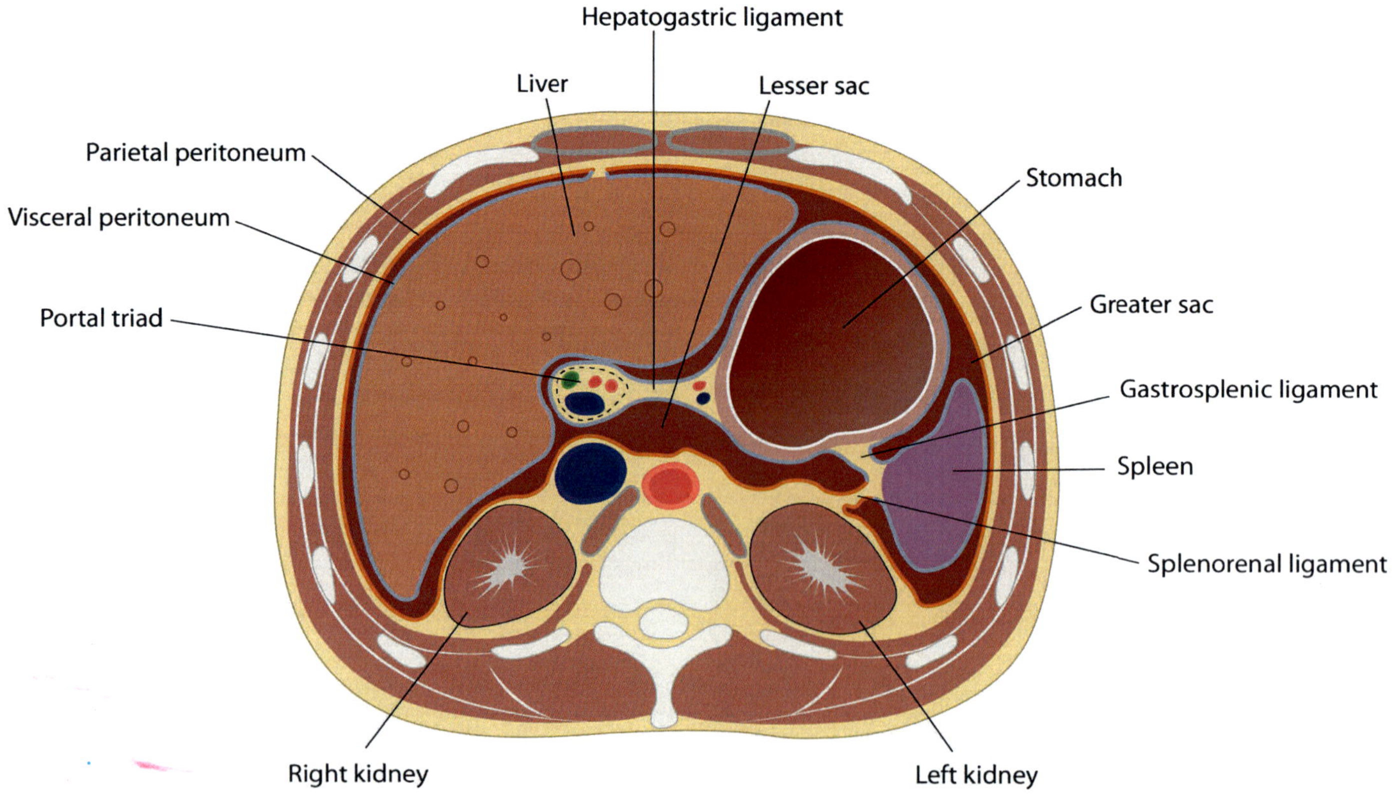

Figure 3.4.3 - Axial view of the peritoneum and mesentery

III. Falciform Ligament

A. Connects to the anterior abdominal wall

B. Contains the ligamentum teres

1. In utero, oxygenated blood from the mother will travel through the umbilical vein to reach the heart of the fetus.

2. The vein closes at birth and is called the ligamentum teres.

3. Portal hypertension forces the ligamentum teres to recanalize and form umbilical varices with the superficial epigastric veins (see Cardiovascular Anatomy Section III - Arteries of the Lower Body)

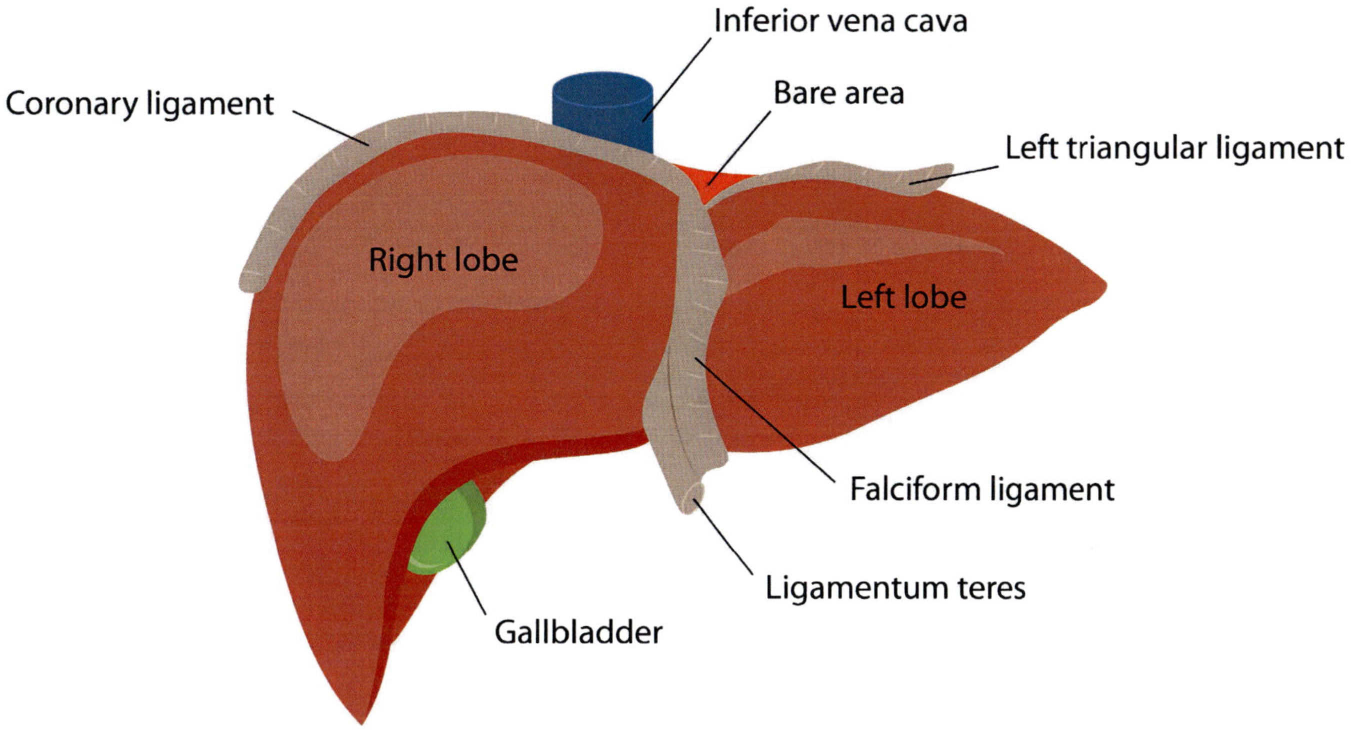

Figure 3.4.4 - Anterior view of the liver and associated ligaments

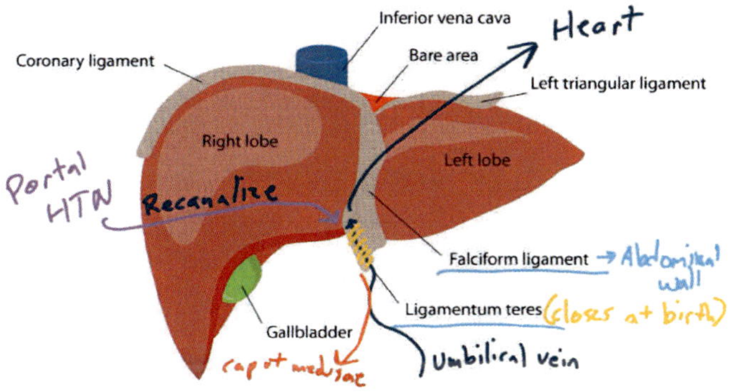

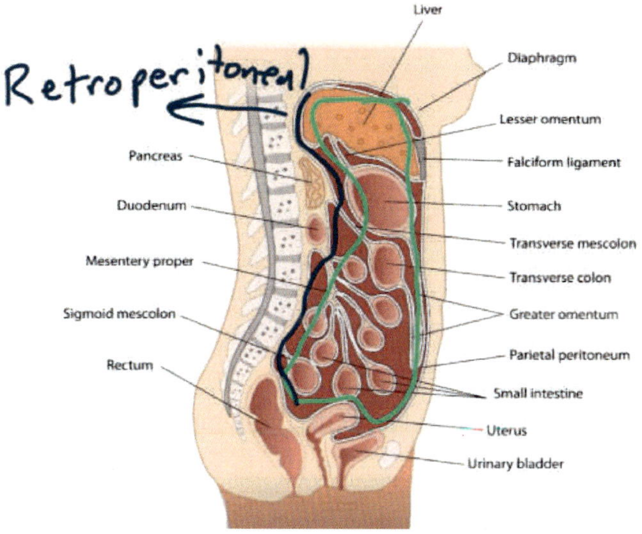

IV. Retroperitoneum

A. Located behind the parietal peritoneum on the posterior abdominal wall.

B. Non-intestinal structures

1. Aorta and inferior vena cava
2. Pancreas, kidneys, ureters and adrenal glands

C. Intestinal structures

1. Duodenum (excluding 1st part)
2. Ascending and descending colon
3. Rectum

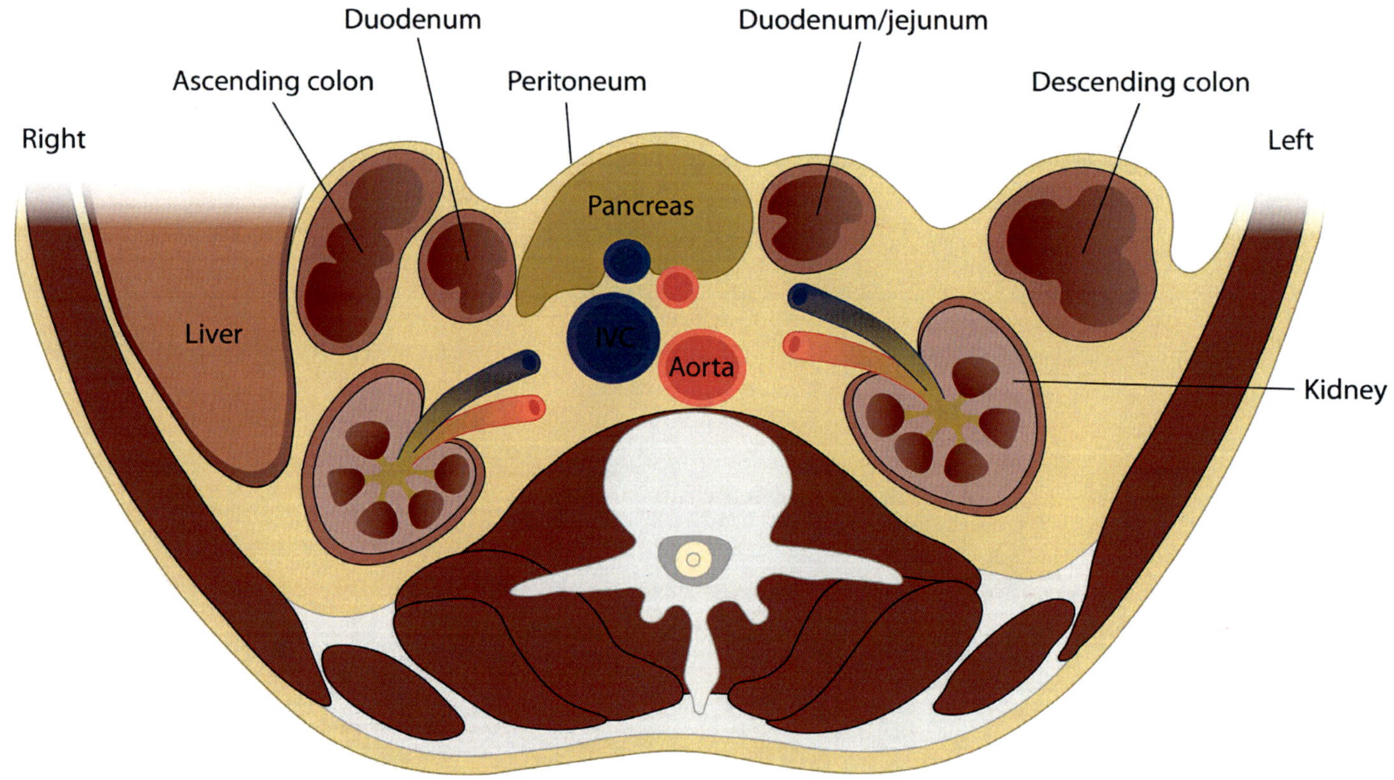

Figure 3.4.5 - Axial view of retroperitoneal structures

V. Retroperitoneal Structure Injury

A. Trauma to retroperitoneal structure → organ dysfunction + hematoma contained within retroperitoneum → compression of IVC or aorta → hemodynamic instability

B. Suspect additional retroperitoneal organs are damaged

REVIEW QUESTIONS

1. An 18-year-old female with sickle cell disease suffers infarction of her spleen during a sickle cell crisis. Surgical removal of the spleen is planned. As part of the procedure, the splenic artery and vein will be ligated. What ligament must be cut to reach these vessels?

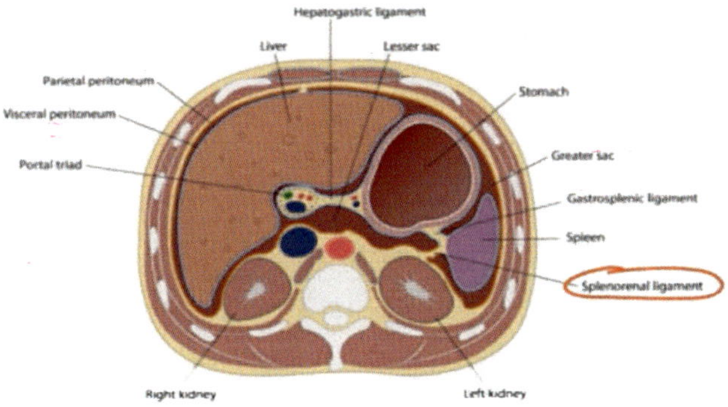

- **Answer: The splenic artery and vein are housed in the splenorenal ligament (the ligament that must be cut).**

2. A 45-year-old male experiences massive hemorrhage following perforation of a peptic ulcer within the lesser curvature of the stomach. He is hemodynamically unstable upon arrival to the emergency department. Emergent laparoscopic surgery is started. The surgeon plans to cauterize the bleeding arteries in order to achieve hemodynamic stability. Which of the following structures contains the vessels that will most likely be cauterized?

    A) Gastrosplenic ligament
    B) Gastrocolic ligament
    C) Splenorenal ligament
    D) Hepatoduodenal ligament
    E) Hepatogastric ligament

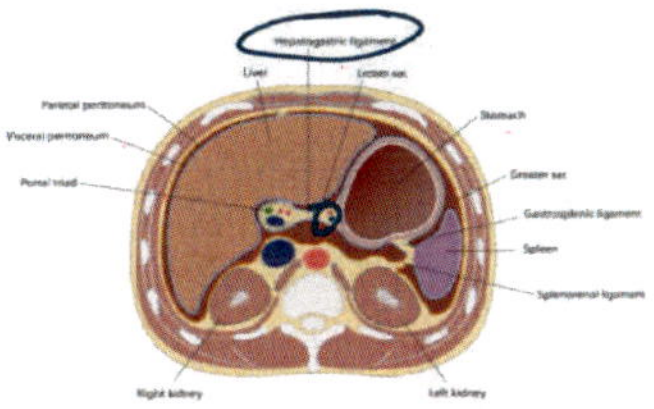

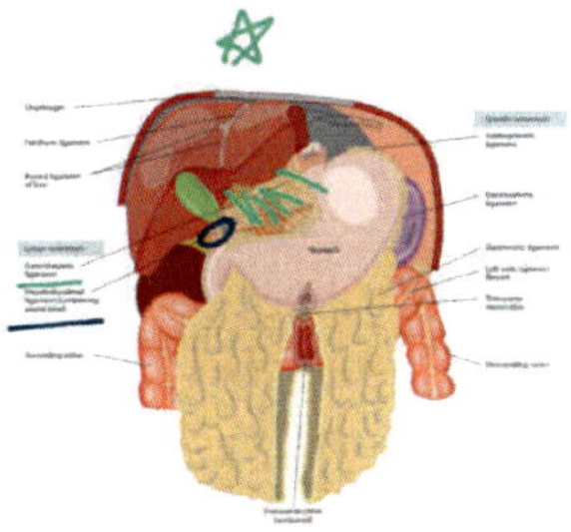

- **Answer: The bleeding vessels are the right and left gastric arteries, which are on the lesser curvature. These vessels are contained within the lesser omentum, specifically the hepatogastric segment.**
    - **The two portions of the lesser omentum are the hepatogastric ligament (contains right and left gastric arteries) and the hepatoduodenal ligament (contains the portal triad).**

Section I.1 - Retroperitoneal Organs

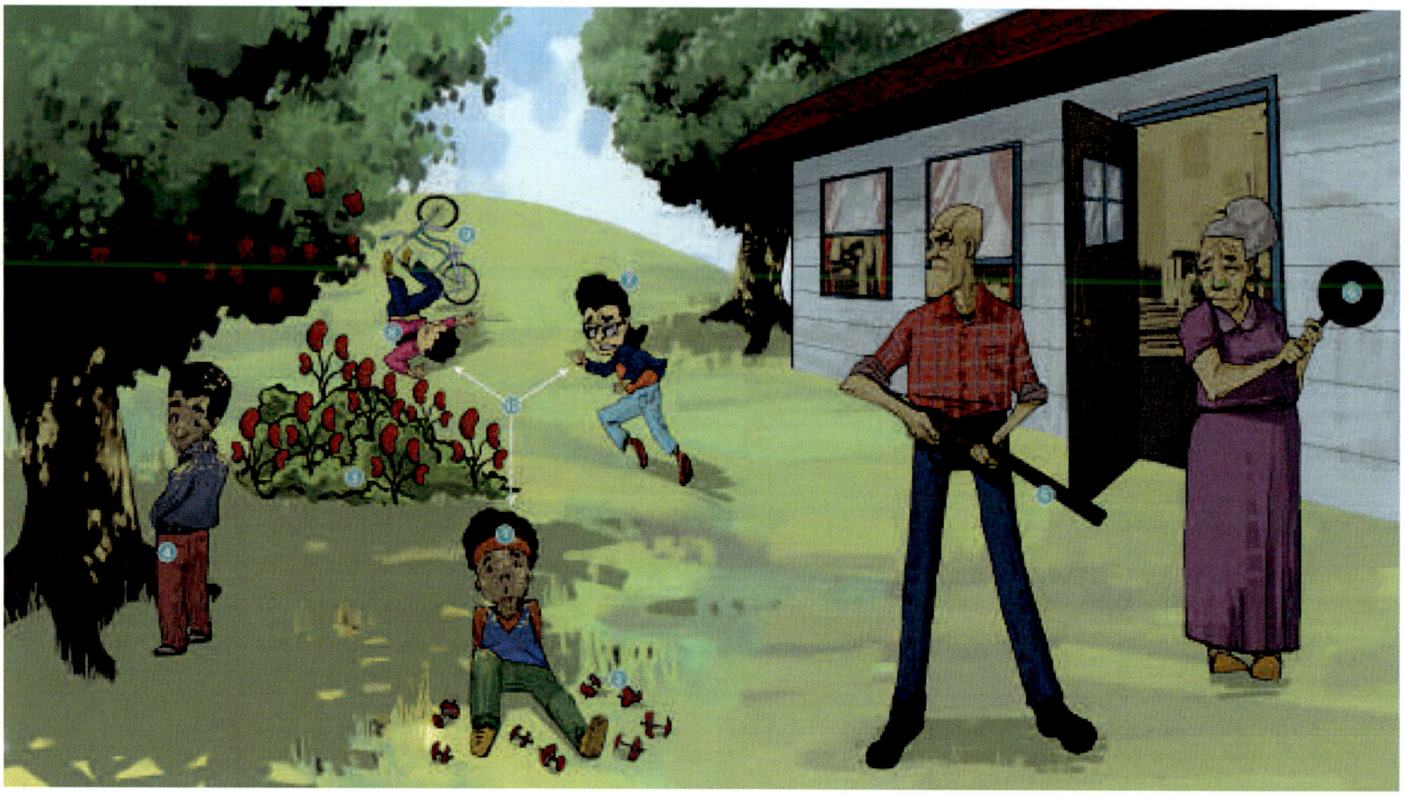

1. ______________________________

2. ______________________________

3. ______________________________

4. ______________________________

5. ______________________________

6. ______________________________

7. ______________________________

8. ______________________________

9. ______________________________

10. ______________________________

REVIEW QUESTIONS

1. A 26-year-old amateur boxer presents to the emergency department following a high-impact punch to the lower back. He describes excruciating pain near the costovertebral angle. His blood pressure is 80/50. Emergency laparotomy is performed. Is the injured structure retroperitoneal or intraperitoneal?

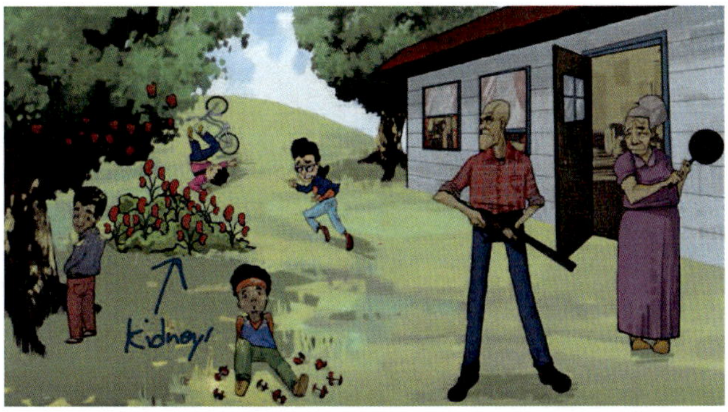

- **Answer: Significant pain at the costovertebral angle following a punch to the region indicates kidney injury. The kidney is a retroperitoneal organ.**

2. A 17-year-old woman is injured in a motor vehicle accident. When she presents to the emergency department, there is diffuse ecchymosis across her abdomen from where the seatbelt restrained her during the impact. She is hemodynamically stable. An abdominal CT scan is obtained and shows a retroperitoneal hematoma. Which of the following structures may be the source of the blood found on the CT?

    A) Distal stomach
    B) Ileum
    C) Sigmoid colon
    D) First part of the duodenum
    E) Internal iliac veins

- **Answer: The internal iliac veins (choice E) branch from the IVC, which we know is retroperitoneal. Choice E is the only option that could be the source of the retroperitoneal bleeding.**
    - **The stomach (choice A) is intraperitoneal, so A is wrong.**
    - **The ileum (choice B) is part of the small intestine, which is intraperitoneal, so B is wrong.**
    - **The sigmoid colon (choice C) is also intraperitoneal, so C is wrong.**
    - **The first part of the duodenum (choice D) should be considered part of the stomach, at least in the context of the peritoneum. This makes choice D wrong.**
    - **Note: Remember this kid who ate too much. "Ate" stands for aorta. If the aorta is retroperitoneal, then so is the IVC and the branches of both vessels.**

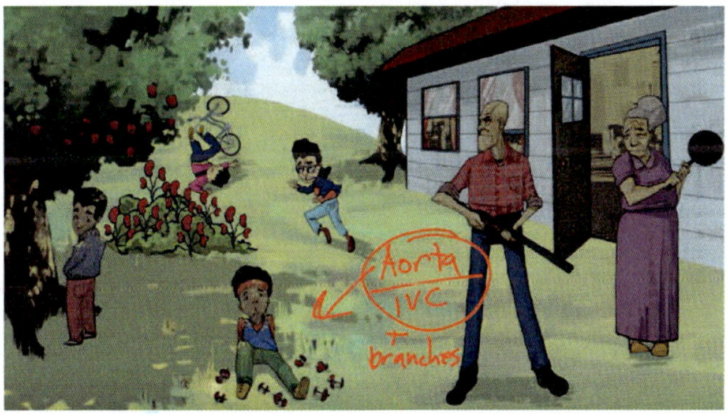

Section II - Inguinal Canal

I. Hesselbach's triangle

   A. The location of direct inguinal hernias

   B. Has 3 borders

      1. Inguinal ligament (inferior border)
      2. Inferior epigastrics (lateral border)
      3. Rectus abdominis (medial border)

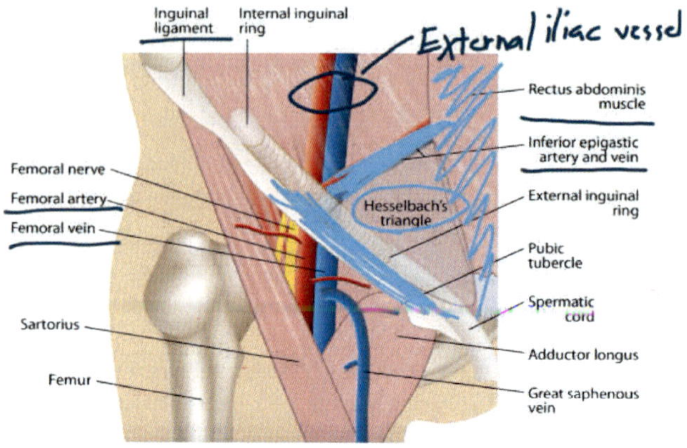

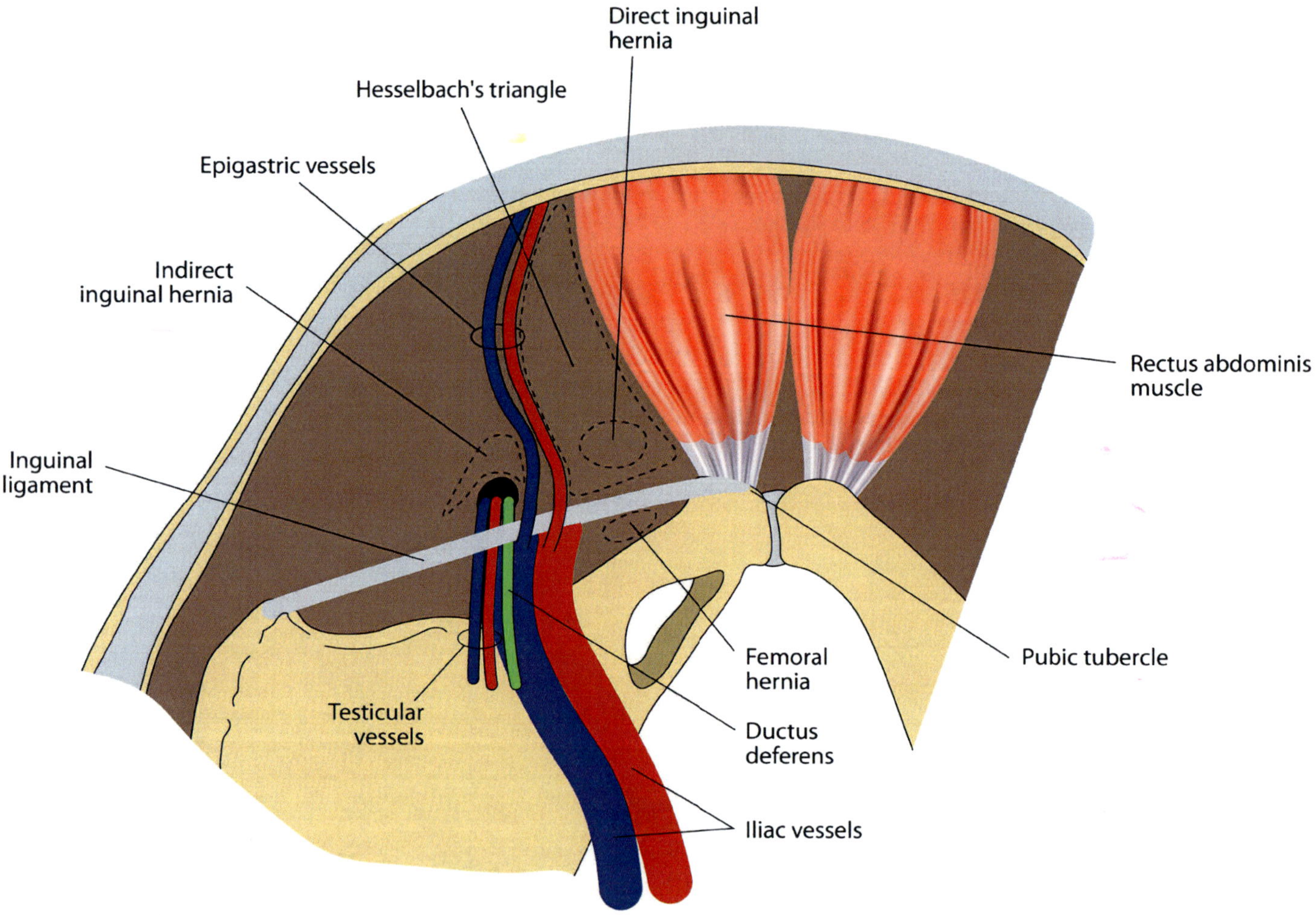

Figure 3.4.6 - Hesselbach's triangle (surgeon's view)

Hernia	Location	Spermatic fascia	Notes
Indirect inguinal	• Protrudes through patent processus vaginalis • Internal (deep) and external (superficial) rings • Internal (deep) and external (superficial) rings • Lateral to the inferior epigastrics	• Covered by all 3 layers of spermatic fascia	• Most common hernias • Men > women • Infants and heavy lifters • "MDs don't LI"
Direct inguinal)	• Protrudes through weak transversalis fascia • External (superficial) ring only • Medial to inferior epigastrics (in Hesselbach's triangle)	• Covered by external spermatic fascia only	• Elderly with weak transversalis fascia • "MDs don't LI"
Femoral	• Below inguinal ligament • Medial to femoral artery and vein (femoral sheath)		• Women > men

Table 3.4.2 - Femoral and inguinal hernias

II. Inguinal Canal

A. Females: conveys round ligament of uterus

B. Males: conveys spermatic cord

C. Larger in males and more likely to produce hernias

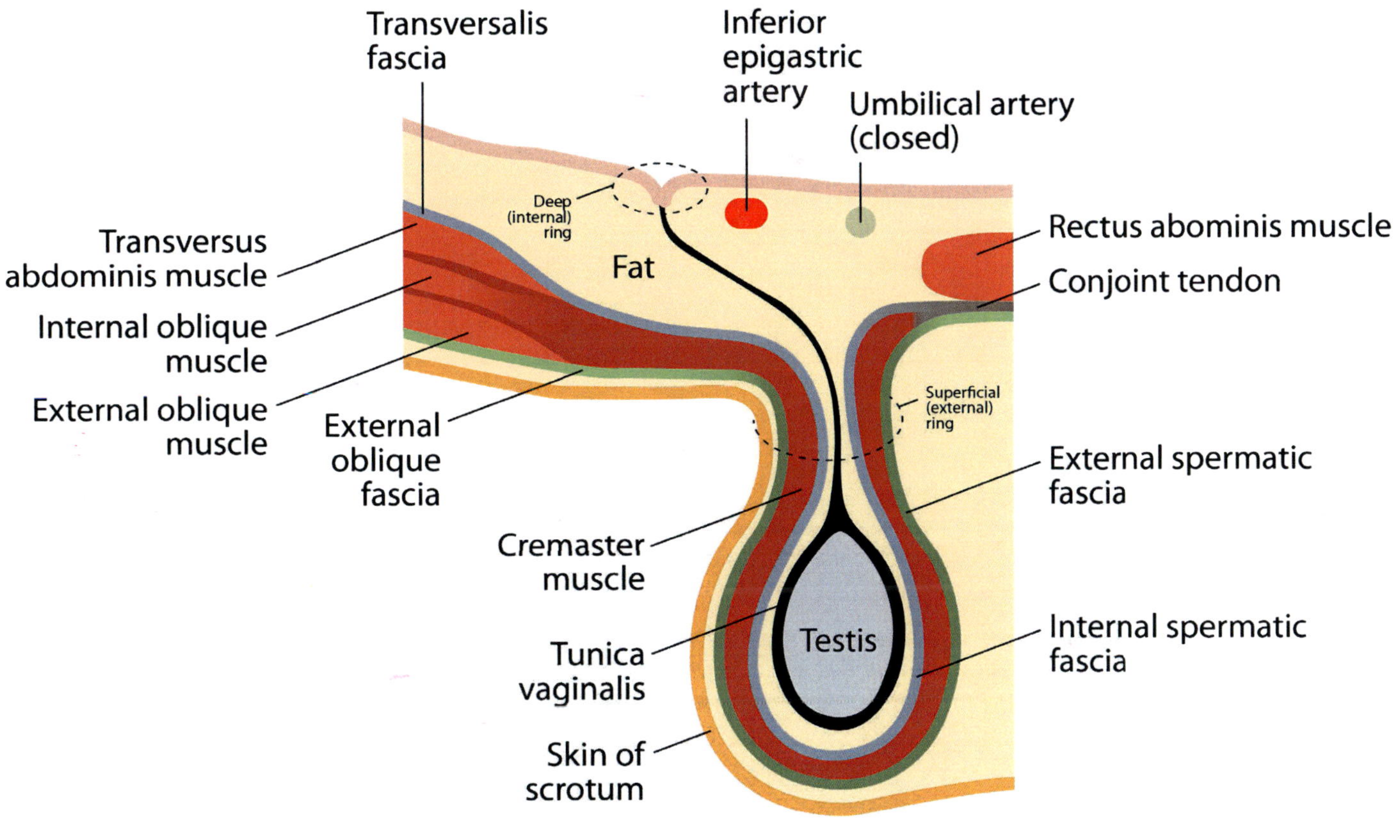

Figure 3.4.7 - Layers of the inguinal canal

III. Spermatic Fascia

A. Has 3 layers which cover the testicle

1. Internal spermatic fascia (transversalis fascia)
2. Cremasteric muscle and fascia (internal oblique muscle)
3. External spermatic fascia (external oblique muscle)

B. Memory hook: ICE tie

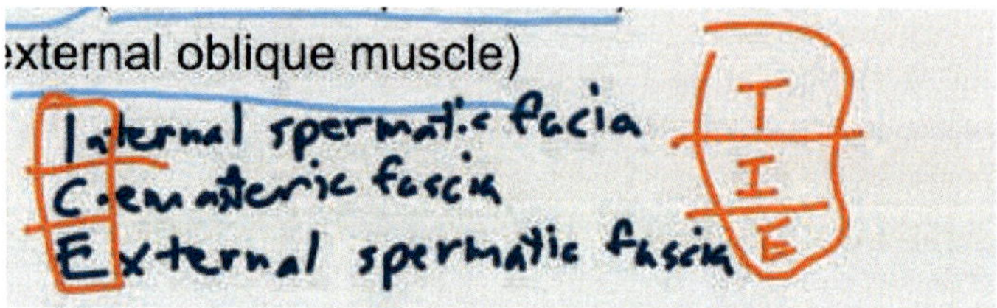

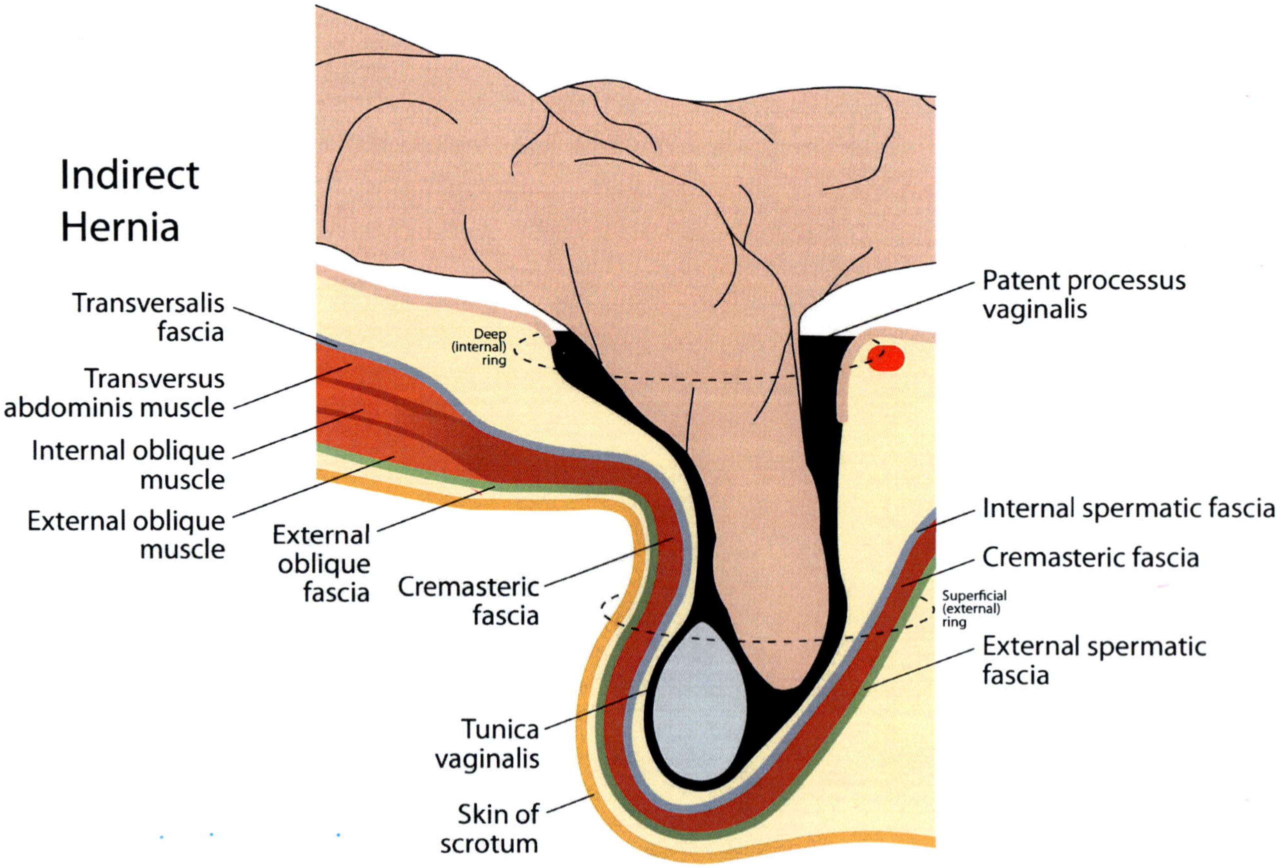

Figure 3.4.8 - Indirect inguinal hernia

IV. Femoral Hernias

A. Occurs when the intestines herniate through femoral ring (medial to femoral vessels)

B. Women > men

C. Note: Even in women, indirect inguinal hernias are still more common than femoral hernias

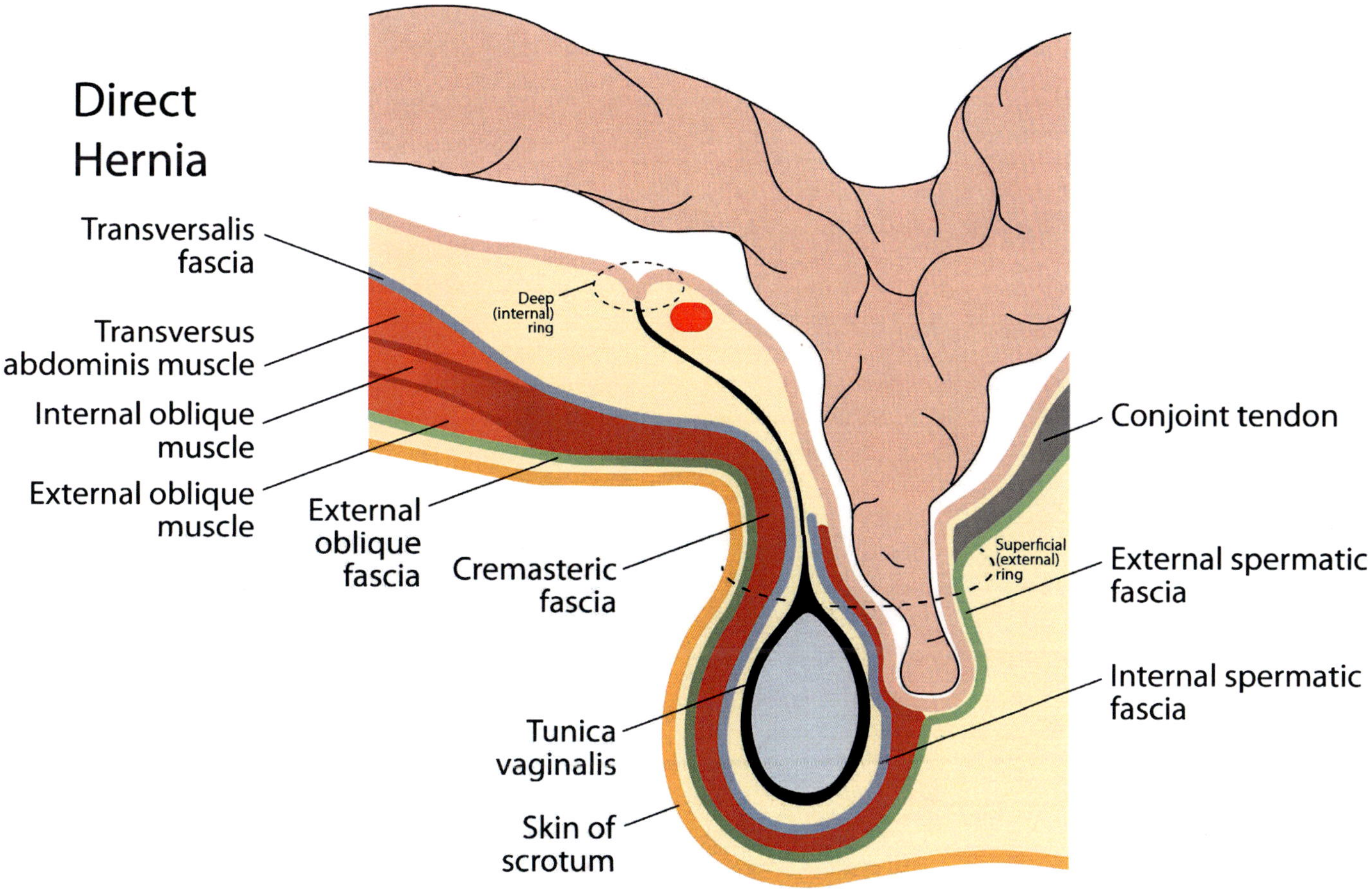

Figure 3.4.9 - Direct inguinal hernia

REVIEW QUESTIONS

1. A 36-year-old obese male presents with a painless mass in his scrotum. He works at a factory that requires him to lift heavy boxes. The first time he noticed the mass was last week after lifting something heavy. The physician palpates the scrotum. From the skin to the testes, what layers of the spermatic fascia is he feeling? What structures give rise to each of these layers?

   - **Answer: The layers of the spermatic fascia can be remembered using the mnemonic "ICE". From the outside (skin) to the inside (testicle) these layers are ordered as external spermatic fascia, cremasteric fascia, and the internal spermatic fascia.**
   - **The layers of the abdominal wall that give rise to the spermatic fascial layers can be remembered using the mnemonic "TIE". Transversalis fascia gives rise to the internal spermatic fascia. The internal oblique muscle gives rise to the cremasteric fascia. The external oblique muscle gives rise to the external spermatic fascia.**

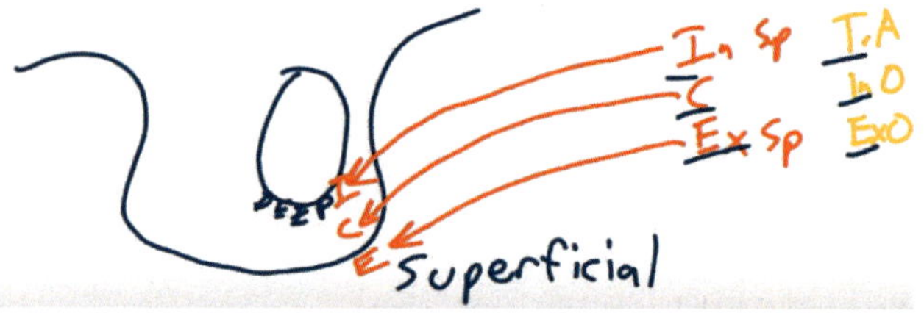

2. A 41-year-old woman is found to have a direct inguinal hernia on the left side. A branch of the external iliac artery supplies the abdominal wall. Where are the intestines protruding through the abdominal wall in relation to this vascular branch?

   - **Answer: Direct inguinal hernias occur medial to inferior epigastric vessels. Remember the mnemonic "MDs don't LI". Since the intestines protrude medial to the inferior epigastrics, they protrude through Hesselbach's triangle.**

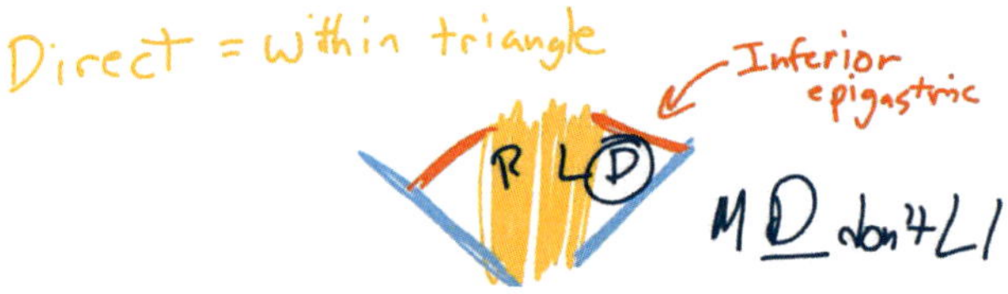

3. A 68-year-old woman presents to the emergency department complaining of right lower quadrant abdominal pain. After thorough evaluation, she is found to have an intestinal hernia near the right inguinal ligament. What type of hernia is most consistent with this patient's presentation?

   - **Answer: Indirect inguinal hernias occur more often in men than women. And femoral hernias occur more often in women than men. However, indirect inguinal hernias are still the most common hernia.**

Section III - Pectinate Line

I. Pectinate Line

   A. Demarcates hindgut (endoderm) from skin (ectoderm)

   B. Innervation, vascular supply and lymphatics differ above and below this line

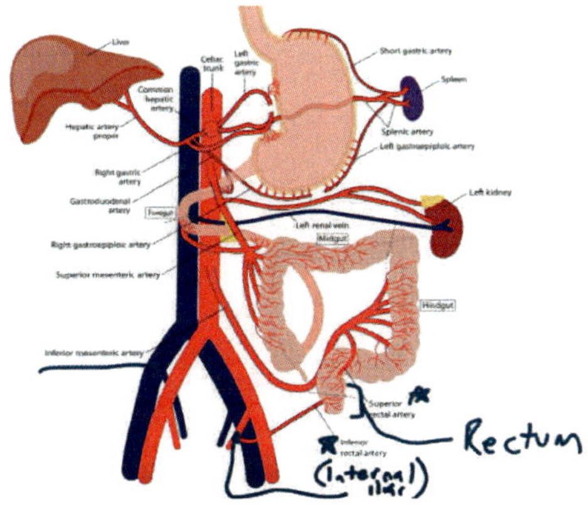

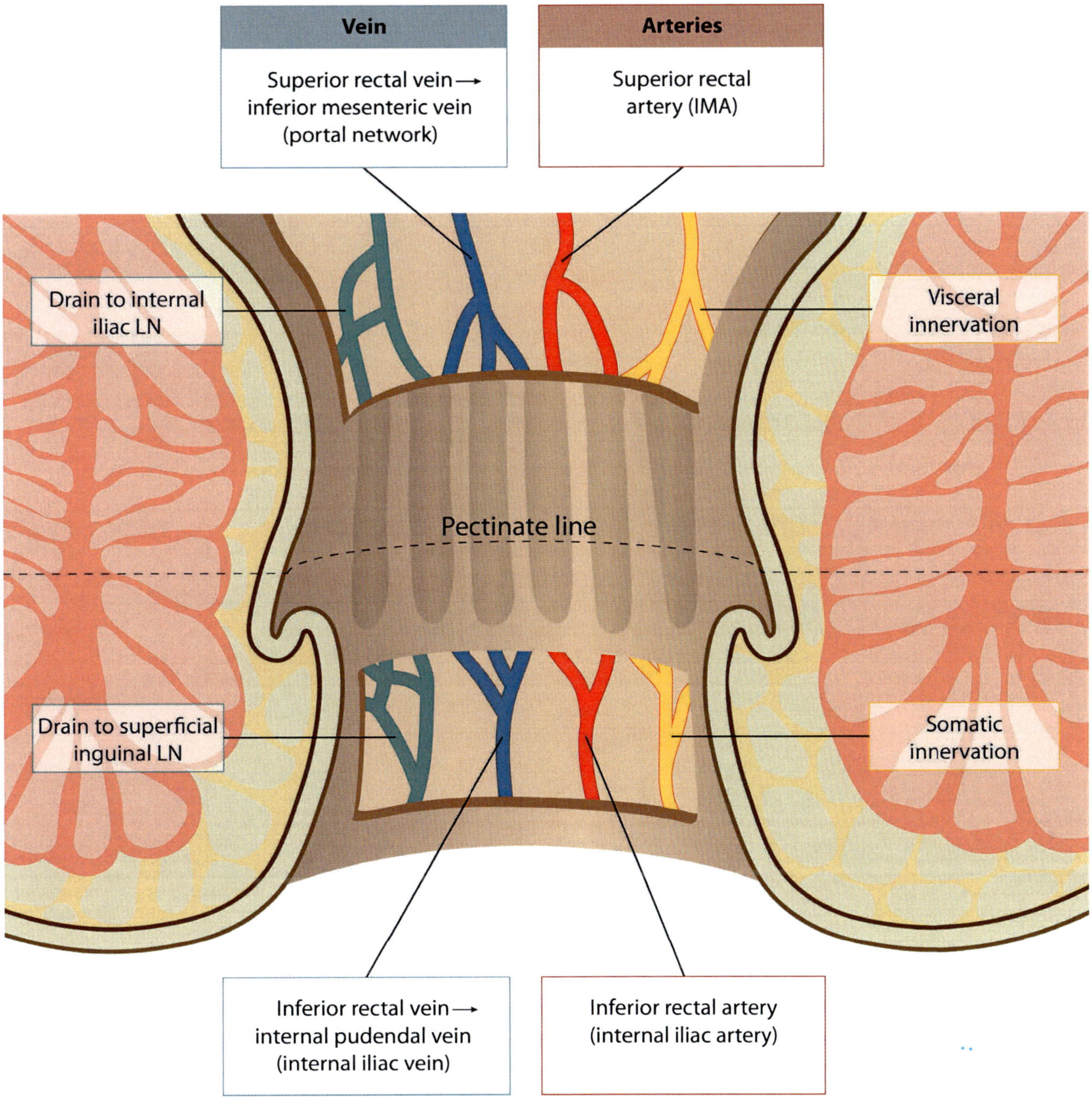

Figure 3.4.10 - Pectinate line

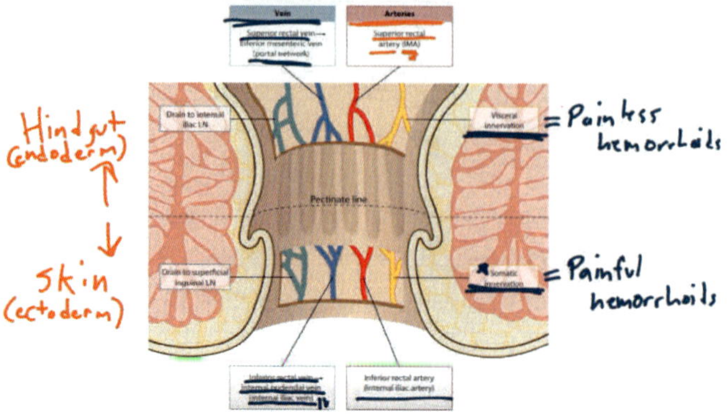

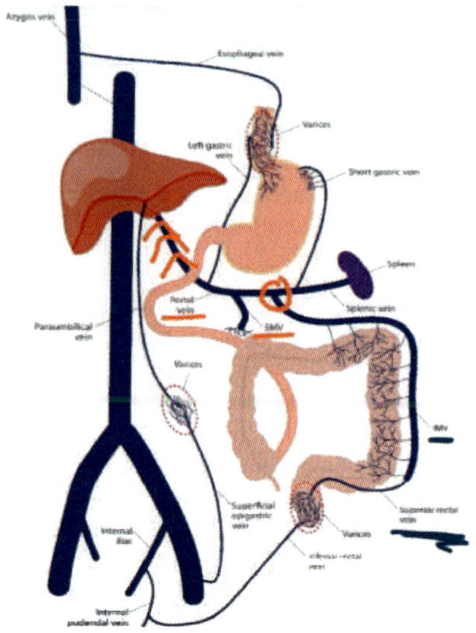

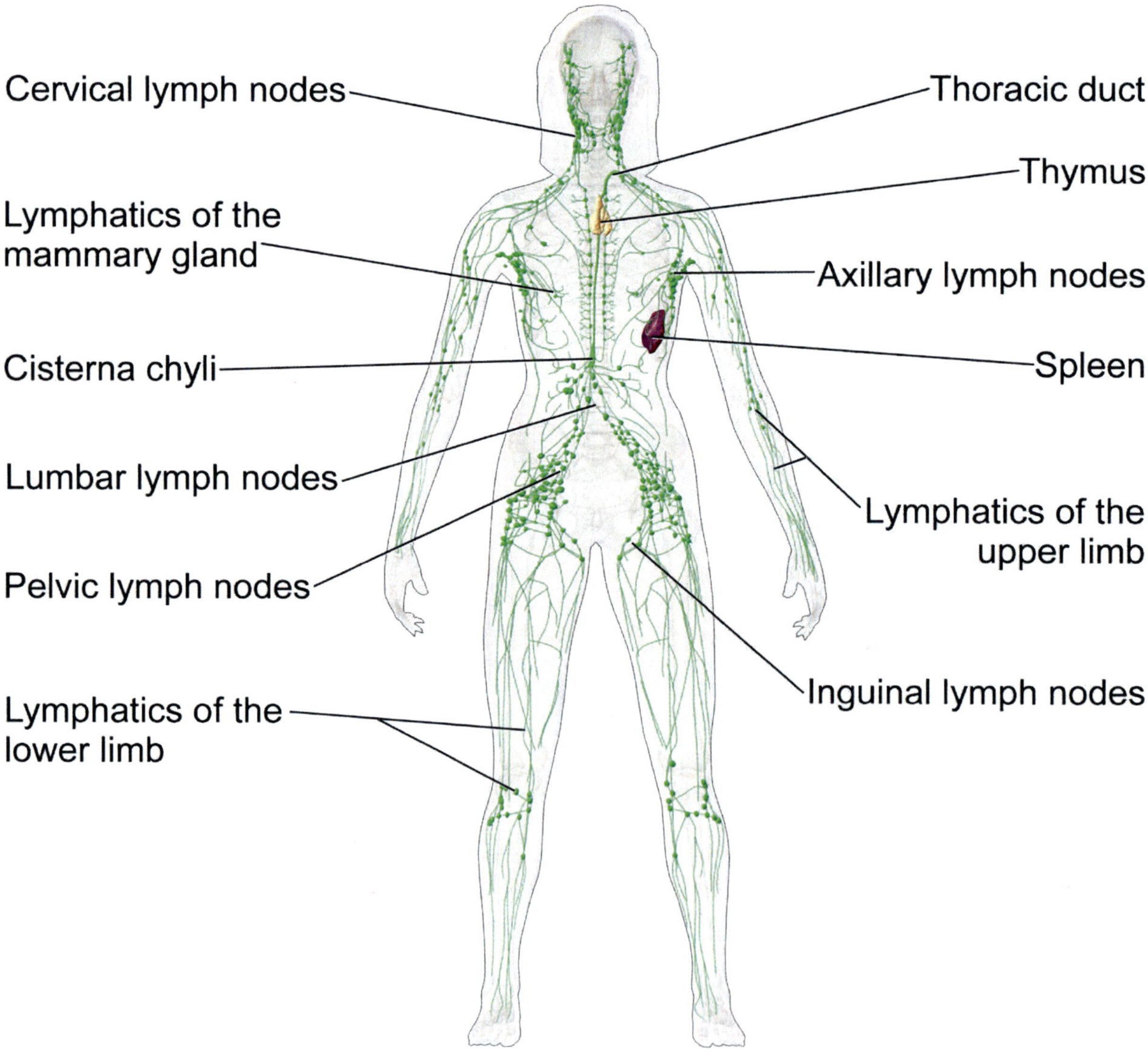

Figure 3.4.11 - Lymphatics Diagram
Blausen.com staff (2014). "Medical gallery of Blausen Medical 2014". WikiJournal of Medicine 1 (2). DOI:10.15347/wjm/2014.010. ISSN 2002-4436. [CC BY 3.0 (https://creativecommons.org/licenses/by/3.0)], from Wikimedia Commons

	Nerve	Artery	Vein	Lymph	Pathology
Above pectinate line	Visceral → painless hemorrhoids	Superior rectal artery	Superior rectal vein	Internal iliac lymph nodes	• Adenocarcinoma
Below pectinate line	Somatic (pudendal nerve) → painful hemorrhoids	Inferior rectal artery	Inferior rectal vein	Superficial inguinal nodes	• Squamous cell carcinoma

Table 3.4.3 - Vessels above and below the pectinate line

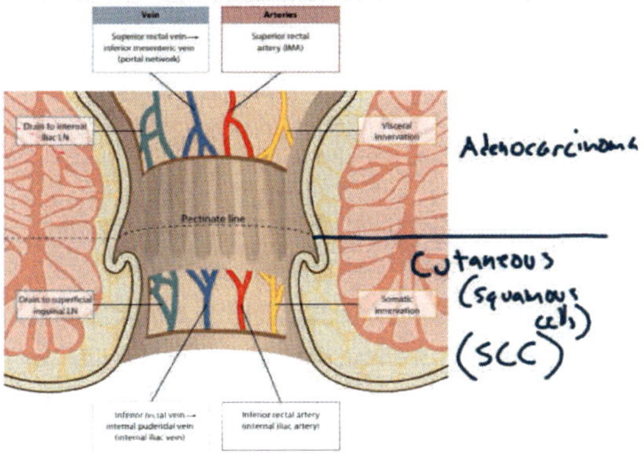

REVIEW QUESTIONS

?

1. A 32-year-old pregnant woman complains of rectal pain during each bowel movement. She endorses the presence of blood on the toilet paper following each episode. Assuming her presentation is caused by a hemorrhoid, the blood likely originated from what vessel?

Inferior recta/vein

Painful hemorrhoids = Below pectinate line (somatic innervation)

- **Answer: These hemorrhoids are painful, indicating they are below the pectinate line, where the rectum receives somatic innervation. Blood to this region is supplied by the inferior rectal arteries and drained by the inferior rectal veins.**

2. A 65-year-old male presents with weight loss and bloody stools. He denies rectal pain but states that defecation has recently become more difficult. He has not had any colonoscopies in his life. Imaging reveals a rectal mass. If the mass is malignant rectal cancer, what lymph nodes will most likely be affected by early metastatic disease?

Painless rectal cancer → Above pectinate line (adenocarcinoma) → Internal iliac nodes

- **Answer: The rectal cancer has not produced pain, making cancer *above* the pectinate line (adenocarcinoma) more likely. The lack of colonoscopies also raises the suspicion of colorectal adenocarcinoma. Lymphatics drain tissue above the pectinate line to the internal iliac nodes.**

Section IV - Layers of the Intestinal Wall

I. There are five major layers to the intestinal wall; mucosa, submucosa, muscularis propria, and deepest Layer. (See Figure 3.1.19 - Layers of the intestinal wall)

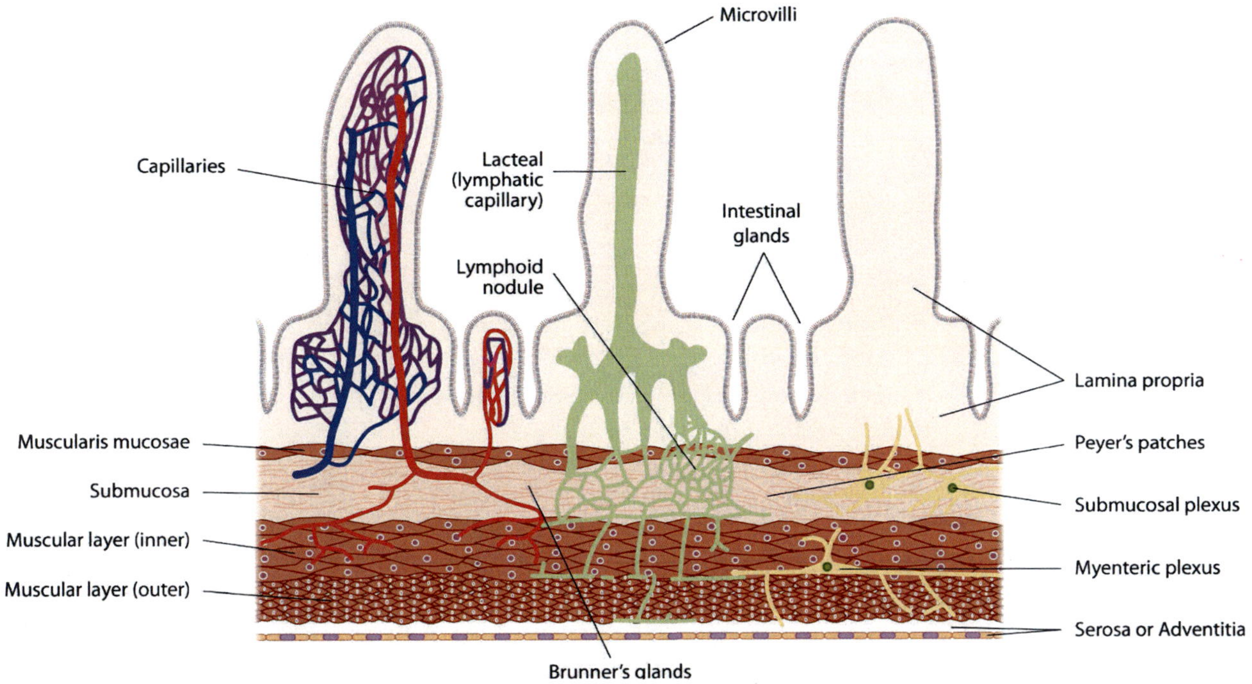

Figure 3.4.12 - Layers of the intestinal wall

Layer	Contents	Clinical Application	Memory Hook
Mucosa	• Epithelium (gastric glands) • Lamina propria • Muscularis mucosa	• Epithelial damage only = erosion • Damage to all 3 layers = ulcer	• "Erode the epithelium and ulcerate the mucosa"
Submucosa	• Blood vessels • Submucosal plexus (blood flow) • Brunner's glands (duodenum) • Peyer's patches (ileum)	• Ulcers reach submucosa → anemia (if chronic bleeding) • Excess acid → Brunner's gland hyperplasia • Infection → Peyer's patch enlargement → nidus for intussusception	• "Pei-pei's brain dump"
Muscularis propria	• Inner circular layer • Myenteric plexus (peristalsis) • Outer longitudinal layer	• Achalasia and Hirschsprung's disease	• "My muscles ache, • her muscles ache, • our muscles ache"
Deepest layer	• Serosa (visceral peritoneum) • Adventitia (loose connective tissue) • Taenia coli (3 longitudinal ribbons)	• Serosa provides lubrication to intraperitoneal organs • Taenia coli can be palpated to identify large intestine	

Table 3.4.4 - Intestinal wall layers

II. Bleeding with ulcers and erosions

A. Bleeding can occur with erosions (epithelial damage).

B. Bleeding is more common with ulcers (mucosal damage). If chronic, iron deficiency can develop.

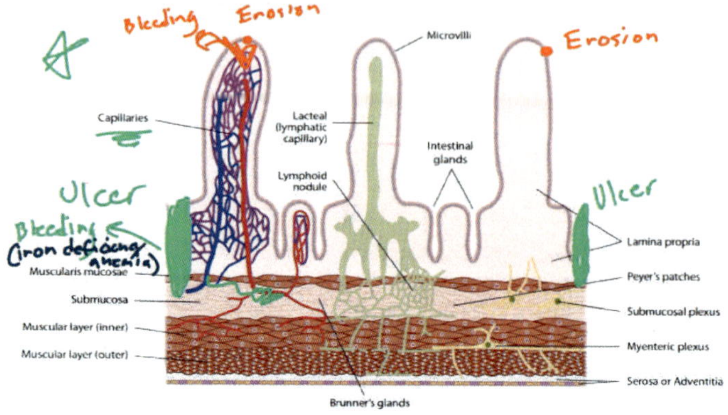

III. Intussusception

A. Intestinal infections can cause enlargement of the Peyer's patches in the ileum. This creates a large object that can be pulled into the colon during peristalsis. This intussusception can quickly lead to a small bowel obstruction (SBO).

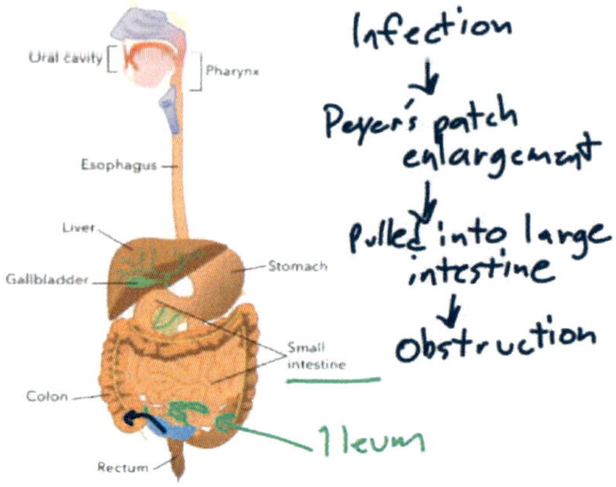

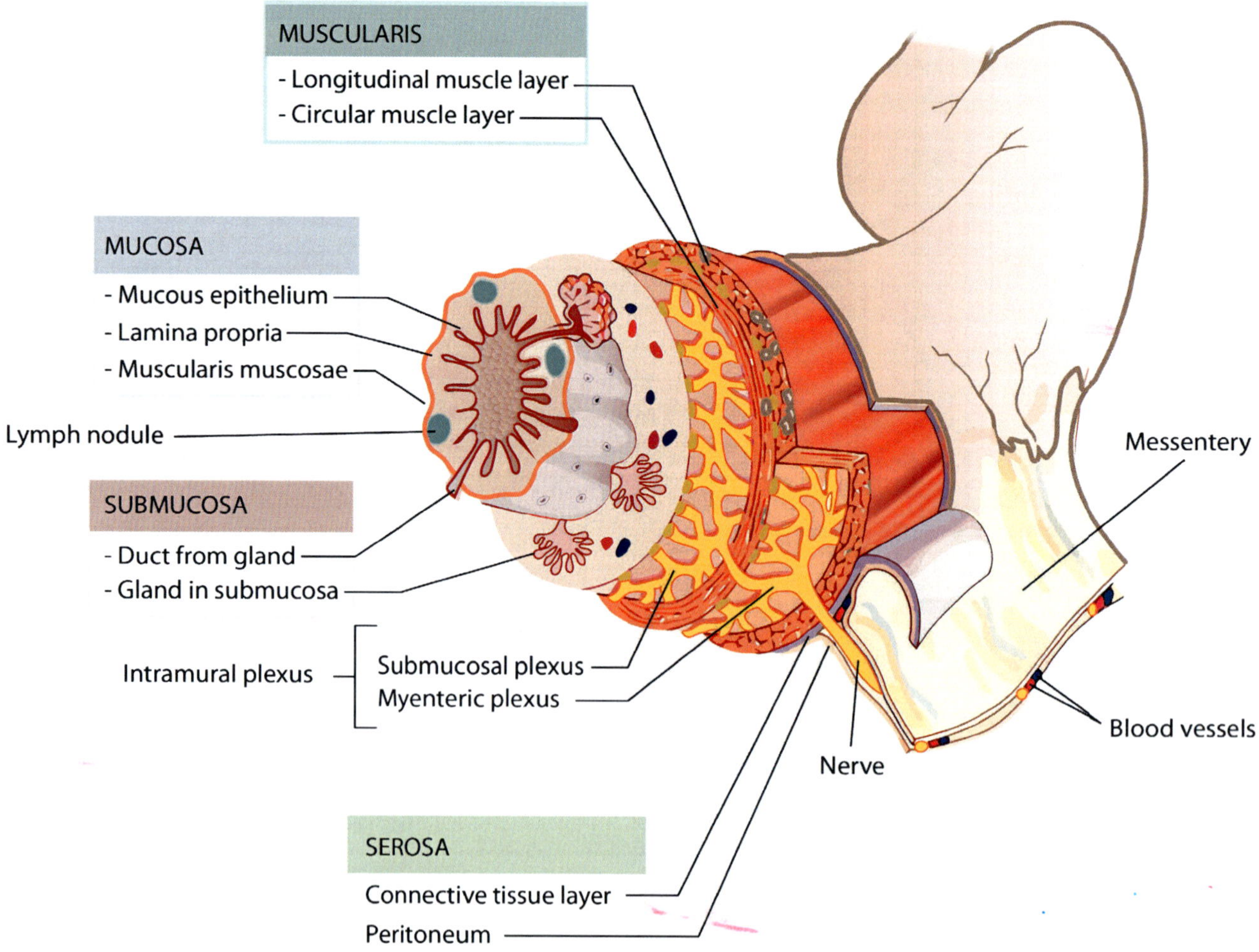

Figure 3.4.13 - Layers of the intestinal wall (cross-sectional view)

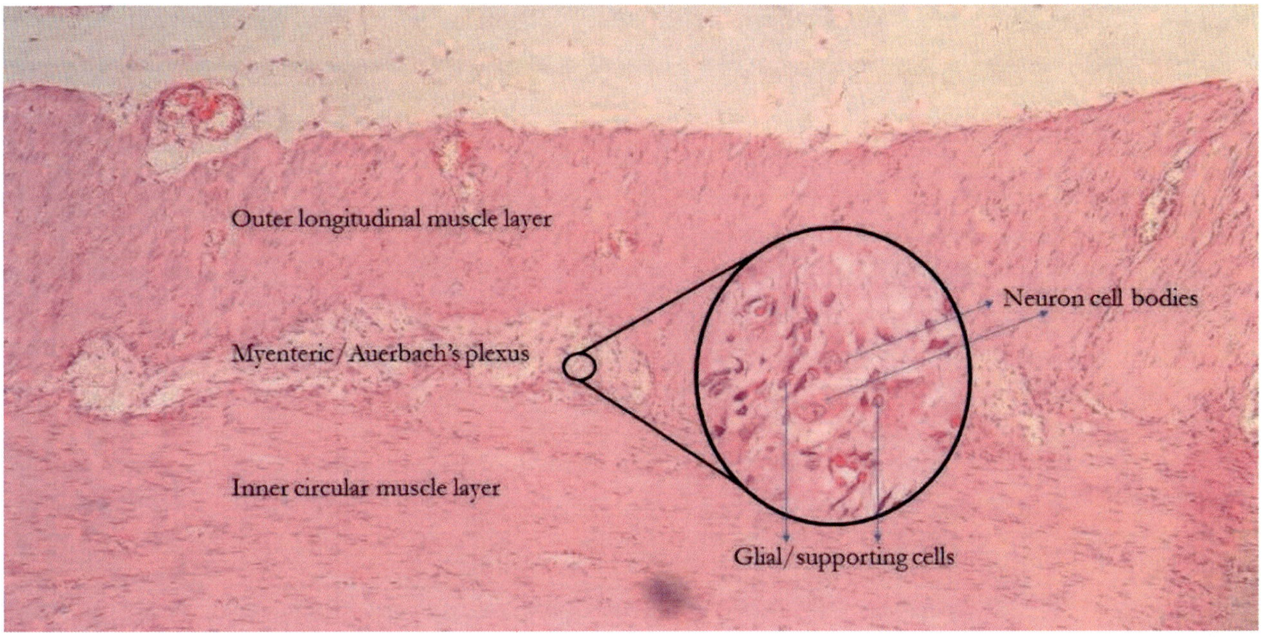

Figure 3.4.14 - Muscularis propria biopsy

IV. Myenteric Plexus Pathologies

A. Achalasia, inability to relax the lower esophageal sphincter (LES), occurs with damage to the myenteric plexus, located within the muscularis propria

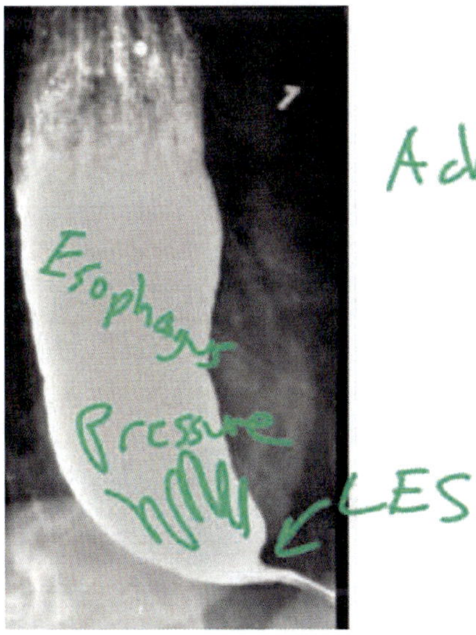

B. Hirschprung's disease, inability to the move luminal contents past the distal colon, occurs with congenital lack of the myenteric plexus.

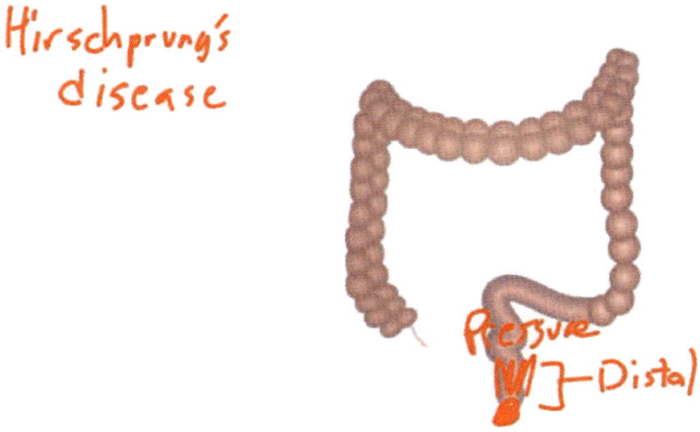

V. Serosa versus adventitia

A. Serosa makes up the outermost layer of the intestinal wall for intraperitoneal structures. Serosal fluid provides lubrication to these free-floating structures.

B. Adventitia makes up the outermost layer of the intestinal wall for retroperitoneal structures. Locked in the retroperitoneum, these structures do not need the lubrication offered by a serosal layer.

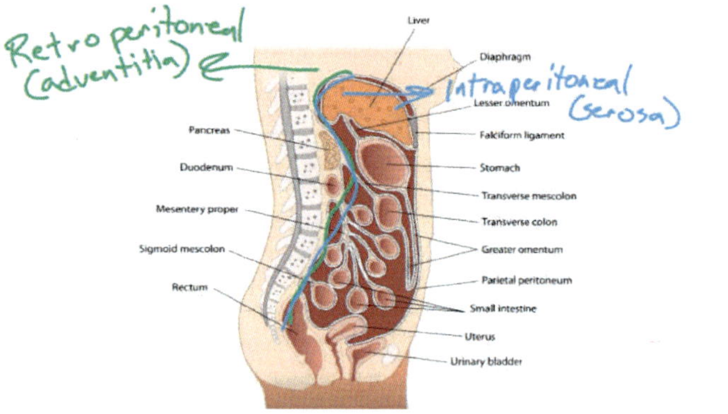

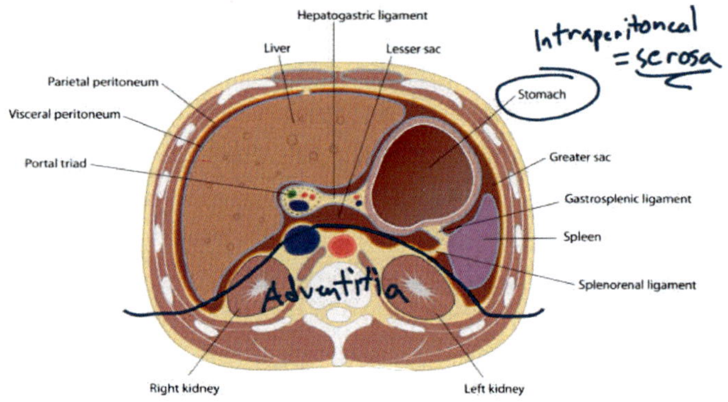

REVIEW QUESTIONS

1. A 46-year-old man with a gastric ulcer is advised to undergo an upper endoscopy. The ulcer is identified and a biopsy is obtained. While examining the histological specimen, the pathologist identifies the cells that secrete HCl. What layer of the gastrointestinal tract is the pathologist examining?

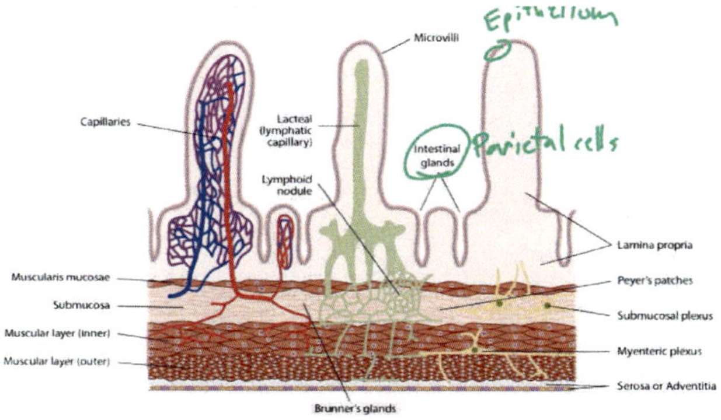

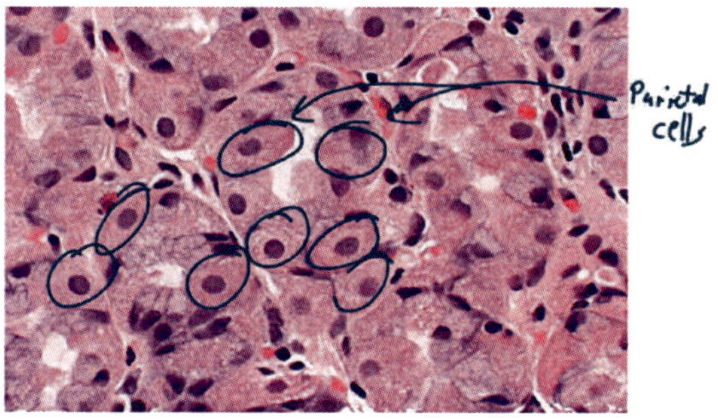

- **Answer: HCl is released from parietal cells. These cells, like most intestinal glands, are located within the epithelial layer. Under the microscope, parietal cells look like fried eggs.**

2. A 12-year-old boy presents to the emergency department with excruciating abdominal pain. A CT scan is performed and reveals a distal segment of the small intestine within the most proximal portion of the colon. The mother states that her boy recently had several days of diarrhea and vomiting last week. If the illness the mother described was the cause of the findings on imaging, what layer of the gastrointestinal wall is likely responsible?

intussusception ← Peyer's patch enlargement (submucosa) ← Infection

- **Answer: This boy's ileum (distal small intestine) entered the colon, indicating intussusception. The recent intestinal infection, as made known by the vomiting and diarrhea, supports Peyer's patch enlargement as the cause. The Peyer's patches are located within the submucosal layer.**

3. A 2-week-old infant fails to have any bowel movements. The pediatrician suspects a deficiency in functional tissue responsible for peristalsis. In the suspected condition, what tissue is defective or absent? What layer of the intestinal wall normally houses this tissue?

Hirschsprung's disease (myenteric plexus) • Muscularis propria
My muscles ache
Her muscles ache
Our muscles ache

- **Answer: This neonate has Hirschsprung's disease caused by a dysfunctional myenteric plexus. This plexus is found in the muscularis propria between the outer longitudinal layer and the inner circular layer.**
    - **Remember the phrase, "My muscles ache, her muscles ache, our muscles ache."**

1. "My" for myenteric
2. "Muscles" for muscularis propria
3. "Ache" for achalasia
4. "Her" for hirschsprung's disease
5. "Our" for Auerbach's plexus, which is another name for myenteric plexus

ENDOCRINE ANATOMY

Section I - Overview of Endocrine Anatomy

I. Endocrine structures include the following:

   A. Hypothalamus

   B. Pituitary gland: anterior pituitary, intermediate pituitary, and the posterior pituitary

   C. Thyroid gland

   D. Parathyroid gland (4 structures posterior to the thyroid)

   E. Kidneys

   F. Adrenal glands

   G. Pancreas

   H. Testicles

   I. Ovaries

II. To understand endocrine anatomy, the physiologic role of each of these structures must be fully understood. For this, see the physiology chapter.

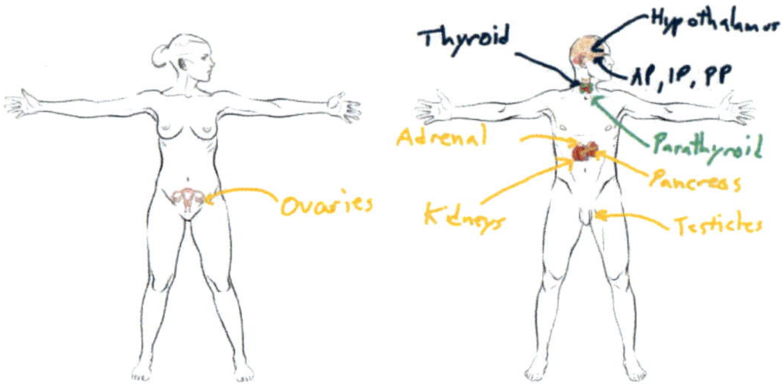

REPRODUCTIVE ANATOMY

Section I - Female Reproductive Organs

I. There are five major structures of the female anatomy that are important for board preparation. (See Table 3.5.1 - Female reproductive structures)

	Anatomy	Notes
Uterus	• Endometrium (mucosa) • Myometrium (muscularis) • Perimetrium (serosa)	• Endometrium grows and sheds each cycle (menses) • Fibroids (myometrium tumor) • Endometriosis (endometrium outside) • Infertility
Ovaries	• Releases 2° oocyte into peritoneal cavity	• Infertility
Fallopian tube	• Fimbriae facilitate 2° oocyte to tube • Cilia to facilitate zygote to uterus	• STI → cilia damage → dysmotility → ectopic pregnancy
Cervix	• Most distal part of uterus	• Cervical cancer • Cervicitis
Hymen	• Circumferential fibrous band with central clearing • Located in distal vagina	• Ruptured during first vaginal intercourse • Imperforate hymen → hematocolpos (blood accumulates in vagina and uterus)

Table 3.5.1 - Female reproductive structures

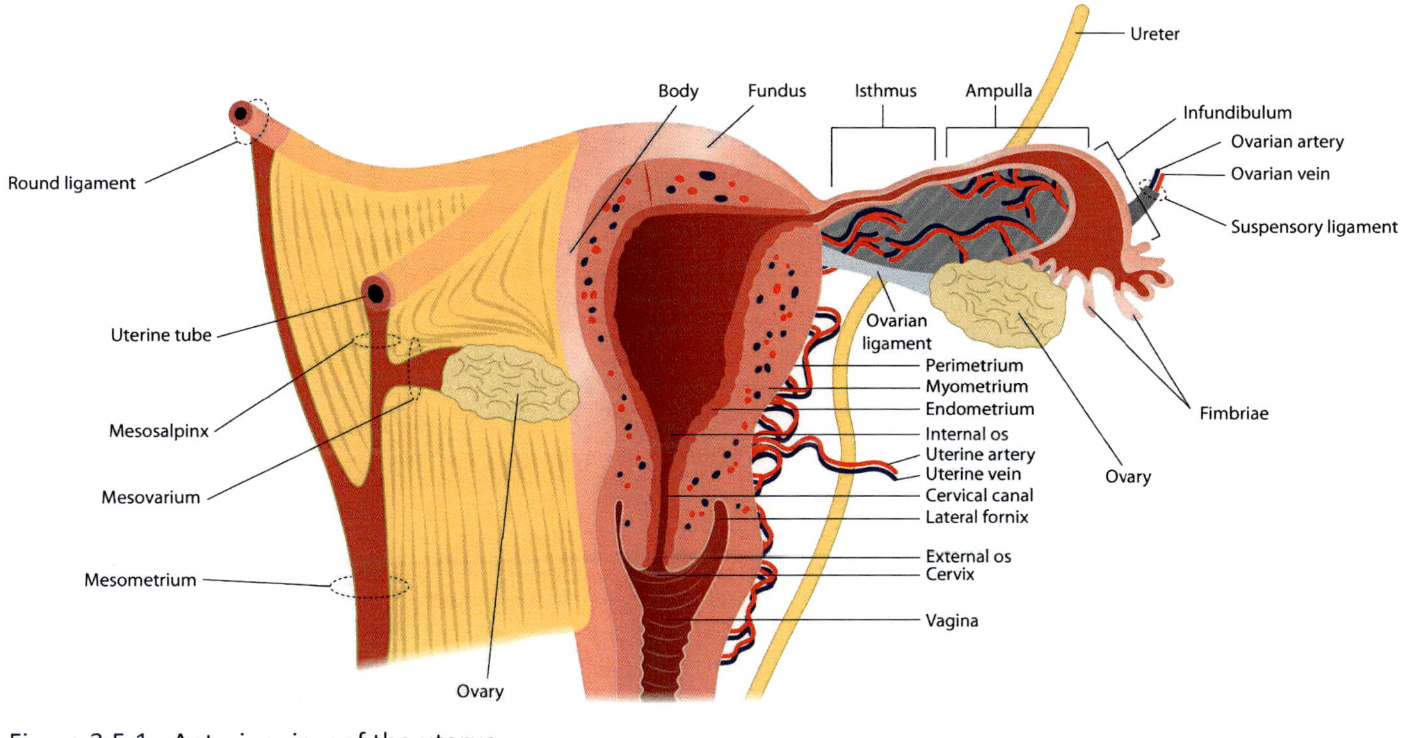

Figure 3.5.1 - Anterior view of the uterus

II. Endometriosis

A. Endometrial tissue outside the uterus leading to cyclical pain

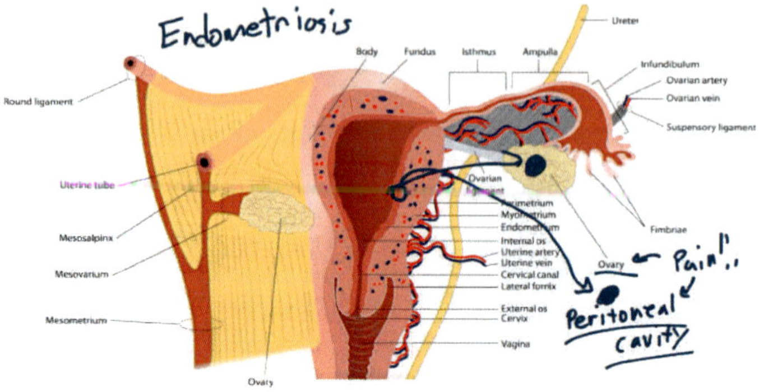

III. Fibroids

A. Tumors of the myometrium (myomas).

B. Can be located next to the endometrium (submucosal fibroids) or next to the perimetrium (subserosal fibroids).

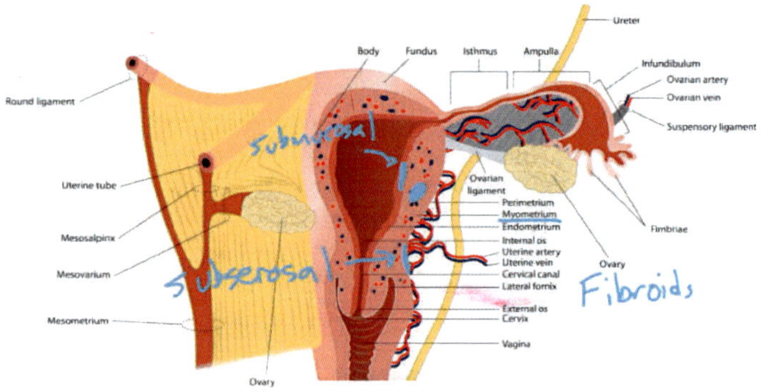

IV. Uterus-Peritoneal Connection

A. Fluid sent up through the vagina can reach the peritoneal cavity. This is because the Fallopian tubes empty directly into the peritoneal cavity.

B. Secondary oocytes get released directly into the peritoneal cavity before being taken up by the fimbriae of the Fallopian tube.

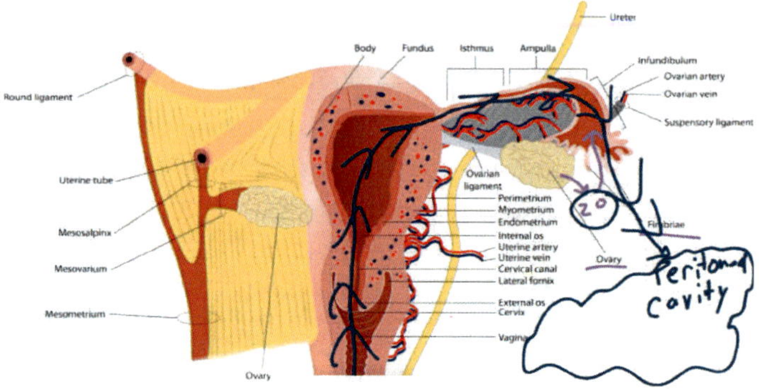

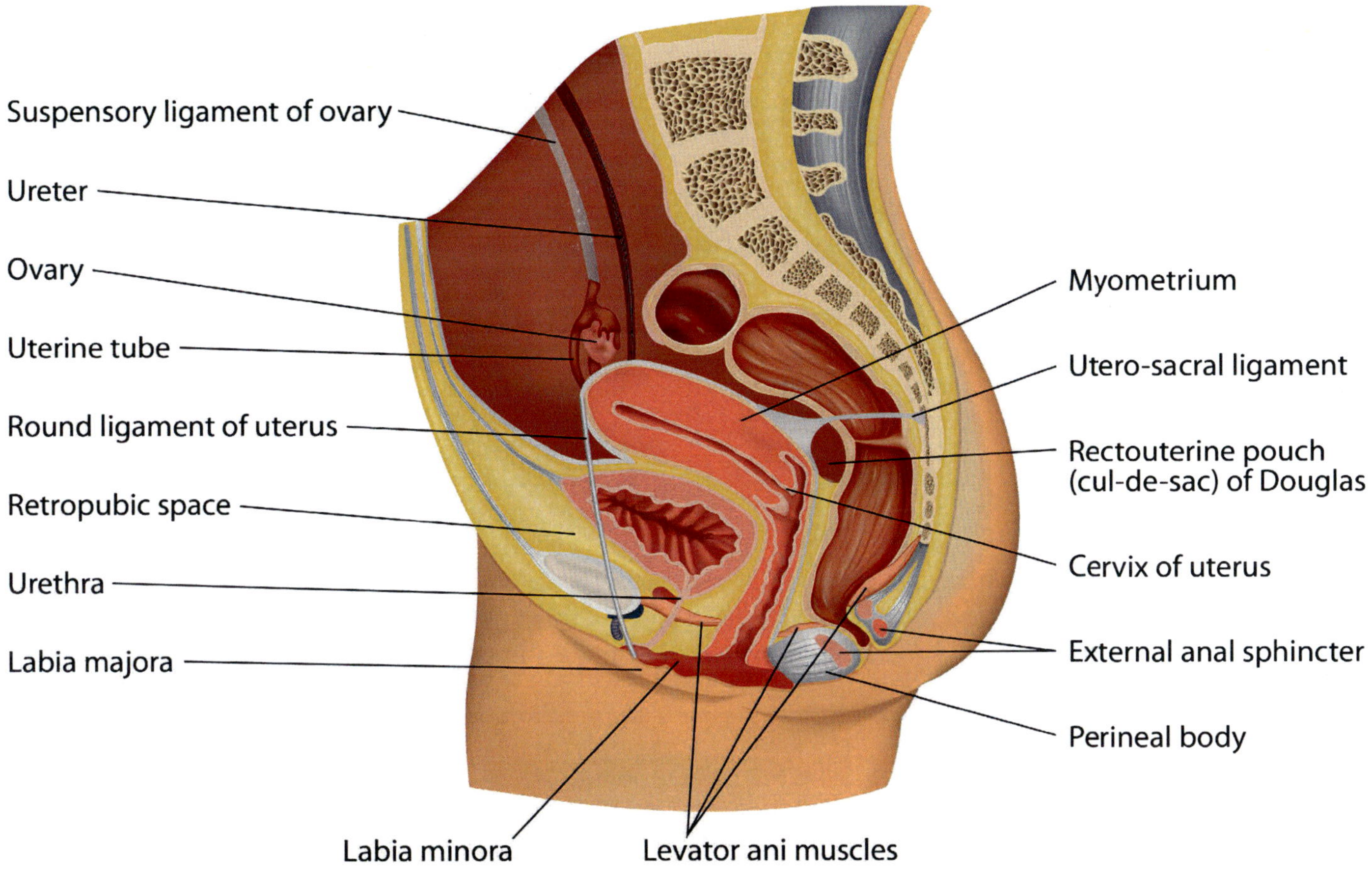

Figure 3.5.2 - Sagittal view of female reproductive organs

V. Imperforate hymen

A. A hymen without a central clearing will accumulate blood after each menstrual cycle. This build-up is known as hematocolpos.

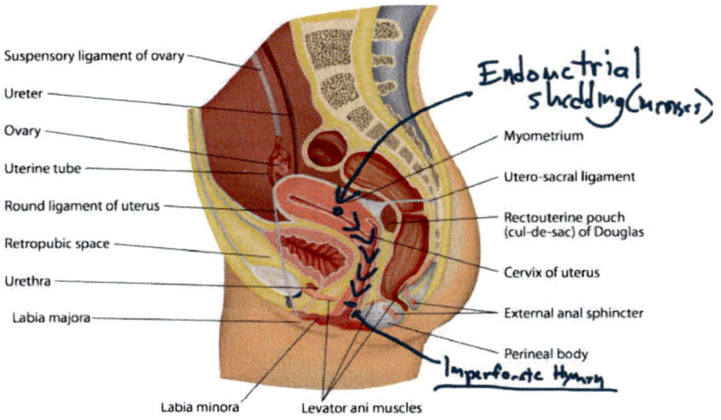

REVIEW QUESTIONS ?

1. A 23-year-old female patient volunteers for a research study. As part of the study, instruments are inserted through the vagina into the uterine cavity where a sample of tissue from the uterine wall is obtained. The sample is examined under a microscope which reveals two distinct histological layers of the uterine wall. What two layers are most likely seen under the microscope?

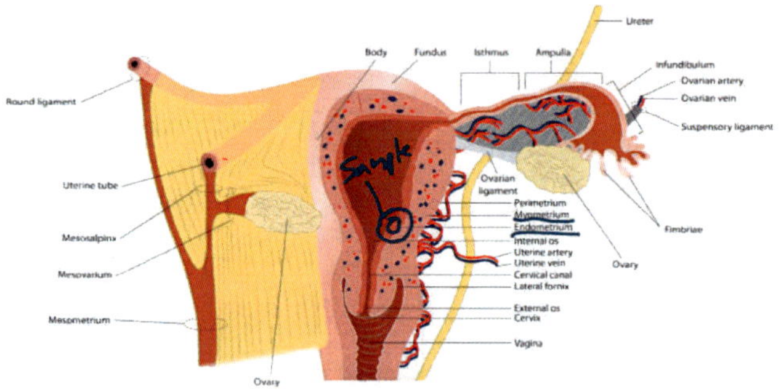

- **Answer: The lumen of the uterus is the cavity within the uterus. This means the luminal layer of the uterus is the endometrium. If a sample taken from the endometrium yields two different types of tissue, suspect some myometrium has also been biopsied.**

2. A 17-year-old female presents to the physician for crampy abdominal pain with menses. This pain has been progressing and worsening with the last two menstrual cycles. She and her partner have never failed to use condoms. Menarche occurred at age 11 and menses have been regular with moderate flow. Hysteroscopy is performed and reveals no abnormalities from the vaginal canal up through the uterine cavity. Which of the following may be the cause of the pain?

   A) Submucosal fibroids
   B) Endometriosis
   C) Cervicitis
   D) Imperforate hymen

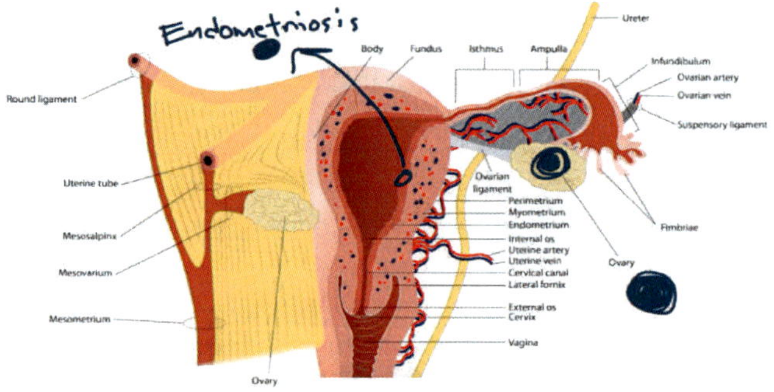

- **Answer: A view from the lumen indicates normal vaginal and uterine anatomy. This fact rules out submucosal fibroids (choice A) which should be seen bulging from just beneath the endometrium. The normal anatomy from this luminal perspective can also rule out cervicitis (choice C), which should show obvious inflammation of the cervix.**
  - **Note: Since she always uses protection, we are led to believe she is at a very low risk of sexually-transmitted infections, which cause cervicitis.**
- **Imperforate hymen (choice D) is unlikely since the hysteroscope was able to easily travel through the vagina. Furthermore, she has had flow with her menstrual cycles, which would be unlikely with an imperforate hymen.**
- **Endometriosis (choice B) is the correct answer since it is caused by tissue outside of the uterine cavity. A hysteroscope is unlikely to appreciate endometrial tissue in the ovaries or peritoneal cavity.**

Section II - Female Ligaments and Local Structures

I. There are six major ligaments in female reproductive anatomy that are important for board examinations. (See Table 3.5.2 - Major ligaments of female anatomy)

Structure	Contents	Local Anatomy	Notes
Infundibulopelvic (suspensory) ligament	Ovarian artery and vein	Connects ovary to lateral pelvic wall Ureter passes posteriorly and inferiorly	• Ovarian torsion → ovary twists around ligament → ovarian artery blocked • Ligated in oophorectomy (accidental damage to ureter) • Memory hook: "Suspend the end"
Uterosacral ligaments		Connect uterus to sacrum (uterine support)	• Ligament damage → pelvic organ prolapse
Round ligament		Connects uterine horn to labia majora Travels through inguinal canal	• Indirect inguinal hernias protrude through inguinal canal (path of round ligament)
Ovarian ligament		Connects ovary to uterus	• Easily confused with suspensory ligament
Transverse cervical (cardinal) ligament	Uterine artery and vein Ureter (posterior)	Attaches cervix to lateral pelvic wall	• Uterine artery and vein ligated during hysterectomy (accidental damage to ureter) • Ligament damage → pelvic organ prolapse
Broad ligament (peritoneum)	Mesentery (peritoneum)	Mesosalpinx (fallopian tubes) Mesovarium (ovaries) Mesometrium (uterine body)	• Transected during hysterectomy

Table 3.5.2 - Major ligaments of female anatomy

II. Ovarian torsion

A. A condition where the ovary twists around the suspensory ligament (aka, infundibulopelvic, or IP, ligament).

B. Compression of the suspensory ligament causes ovarian ischemia due to decreased flow through the ovarian artery

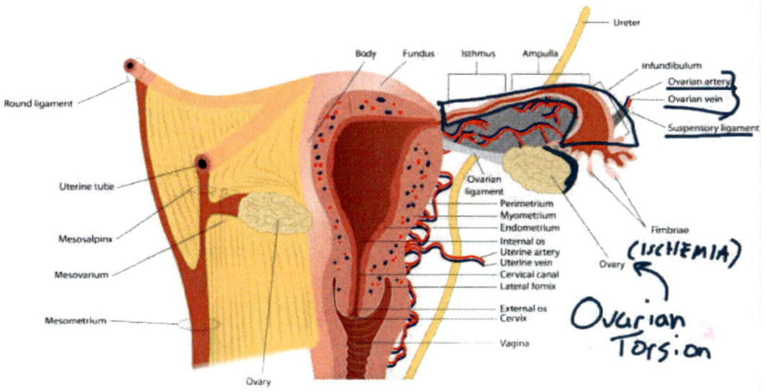

III. The Suspensory Ligament

A. Attaches to the lateral ends of the ovaries and suspends the ovaries by connecting them to the lateral abdominal wall.

B. See more details about the suspensory ligament from the table above.

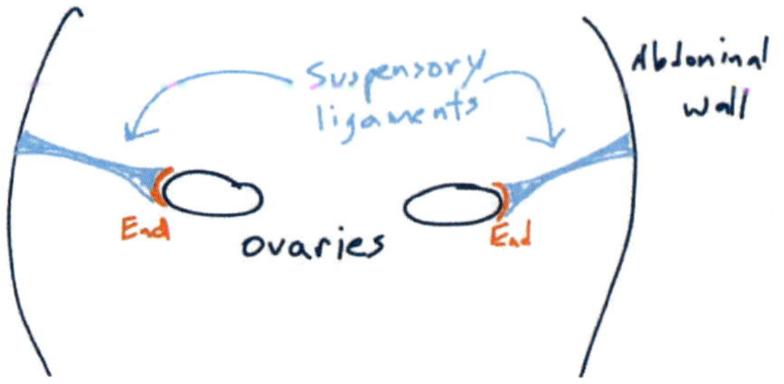

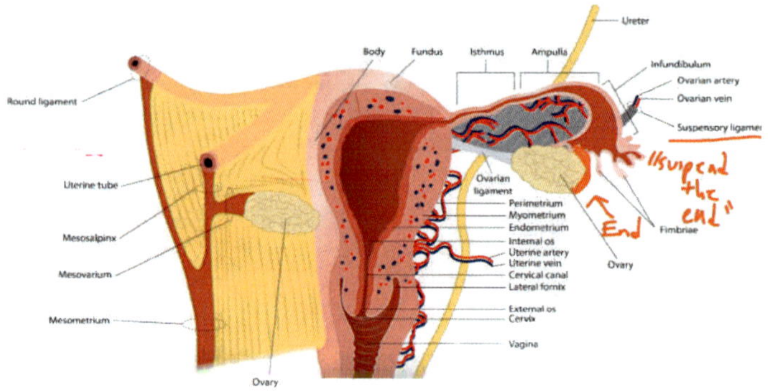

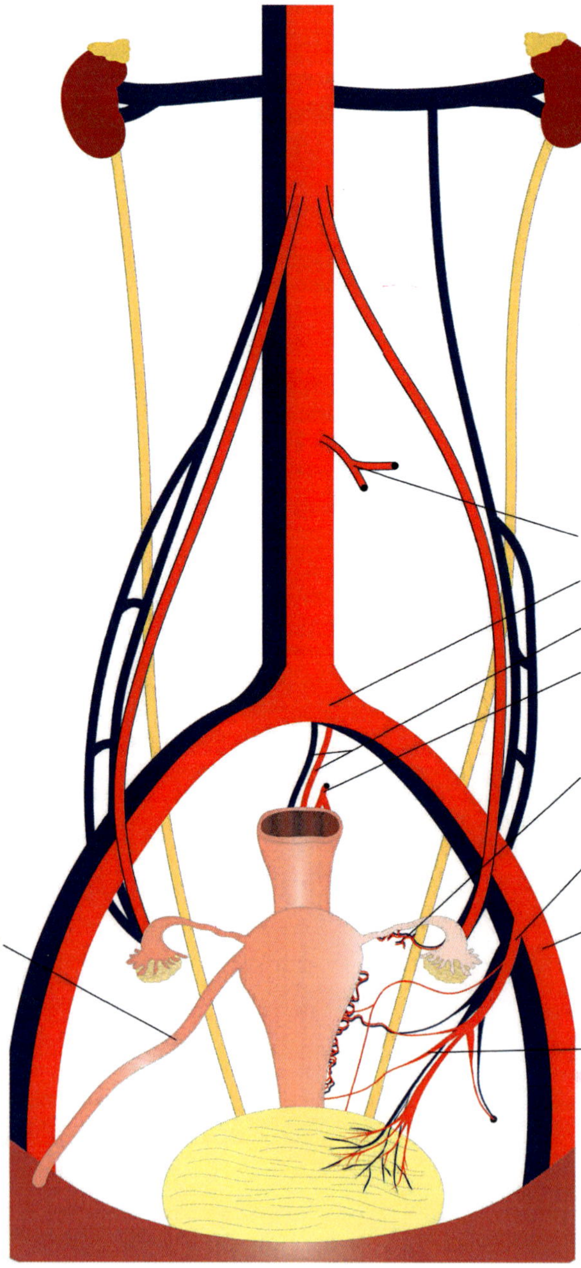

Figure 3.5.3 - Ureters in relation to female anatomy

IV. Pelvic Organ Prolapse

A. Loss of supporting structures → pelvic organs herniate into vaginal wall

B. Supporting structures

1. Uterosacral ligament
2. Transverse cervical (cardinal) ligament
3. Levator ani muscles

C. Urethral sphincter involvement → stress incontinence

1. This item is discussed in more detail in Section III - Pelvic Floor.

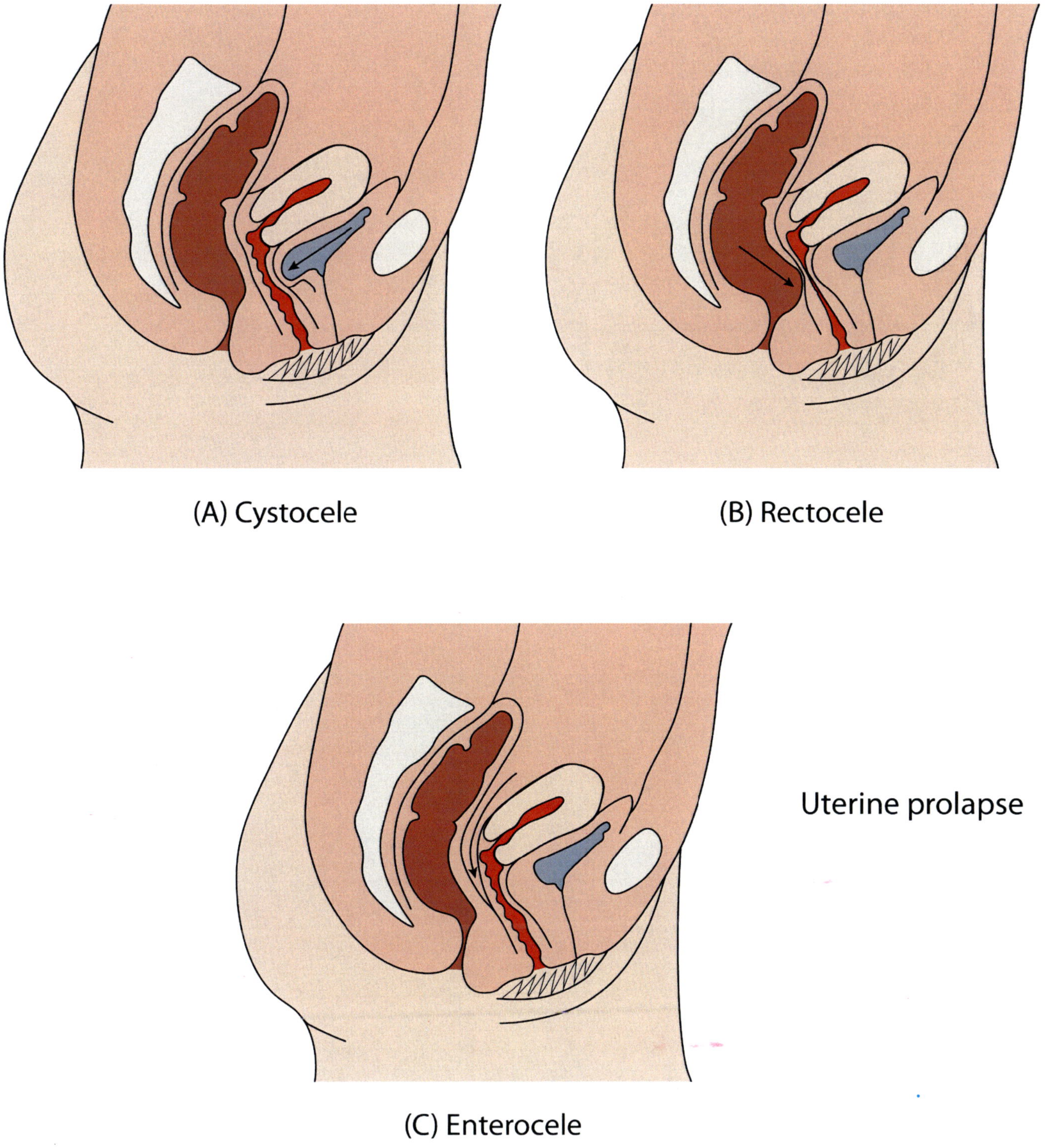

Figure 3.5.4 - Pelvic organ prolapse

V. Transverse Cervical (Cardinal) Ligament Versus Broad Ligament

A. Transverse cervical ligament

1. Attaches to the uterus, at the level of the cervix, connecting it to the lateral pelvic wall.
2. Contains the uterine artery and vein.

B. Broad ligament

1. Attaches to the uterus above the level of the cervix.
2. Technically mesentery.
3. Contains distal portions of the uterine artery and vein.

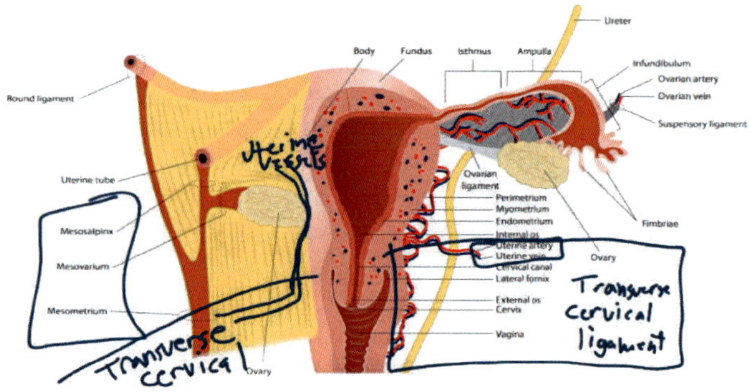

REVIEW QUESTIONS

1. A 67-year-old female presents for a routine physical exam. The physician examines the pelvis and notes that the posterior vaginal wall appears to bulge, especially when the patient coughs. What structure is more likely damaged (the uterosacral ligaments or suspensory ligaments)?

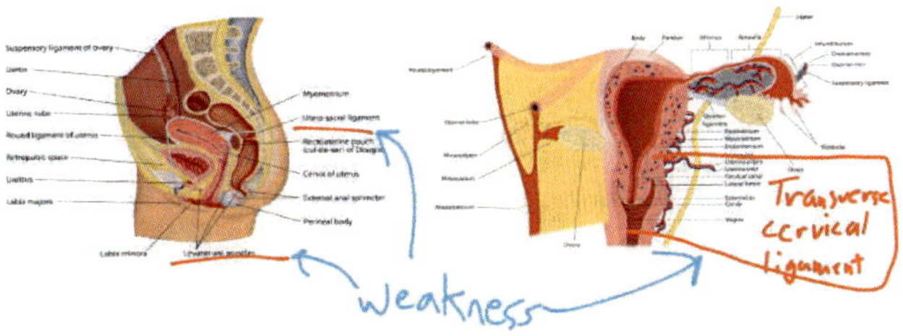

- **Answer: The bulging posterior vaginal wall indicates pelvic organ prolapse, most noticeable with increased abdominal pressure (e.g. coughing). The uterosacral ligaments, not the suspensory ligaments, are responsible for supporting the uterus.**

2. A 49-year-old female is diagnosed with stage I left-sided ovarian cancer. During the surgery, several ligaments are transected to remove the ovary. Immediately upon removal of the ovary, the surgeons see profuse hemorrhage from one of the transected ligaments. The surgeon promptly begins to tie-off the involved vessels. What vessels and ligament is he targeting?

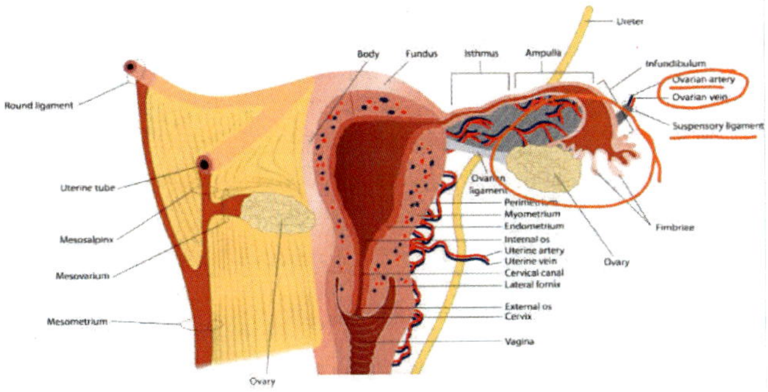

- **Answer: The transected vessels were likely the ovarian artery and vein. These vessels are contained within the suspensory, or IP, ligament.**

3. A 33-year-old female with endometriosis undergoes elective hysterectomy. During the surgery, the physician identifies the ureters on both sides of the uterus. She avoids ureter damage until she ligates the uterine artery on the right side. What ligament was she likely transecting at the time of ureter damage? With respect to the uterine artery, did the surgeon transect too far anteriorly or posteriorly?

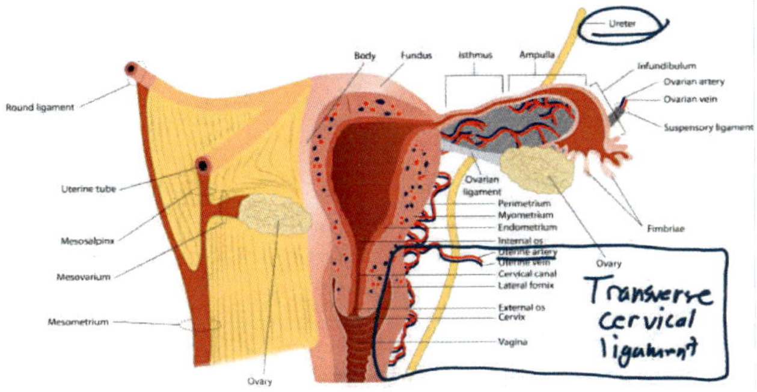

- **Answer: The uterine artery was damaged at the same time as the ureter. The ligament that contains both of these structures is the transverse cervical (cardinal) ligament.**
- **The ureter passes behind the uterine artery and vein, so the surgeon must have transected too far posteriorly.**

Section III - Pelvic Floor

I. There are five major structures to be familiar with regarding the pelvic floor. (See Table 3.5.3 - Pelvic floor structures)

Structure	Anatomy	Clinical Significance
Urethral sphincters	• Internal (smooth muscle; involuntary) • External (skeletal muscle; voluntary)	• Pelvic organ prolapse (cystocele) → weak urethral sphincters → stress incontinence
Anal sphincter	• Surrounds anus	• Pelvic organ prolapse (rectocele) → weak anal sphincter → fecal incontinence (rare) or constipation
Levator ani muscles	• Located on pelvic floor • Supports pelvic organs	• Damage → pelvic organ prolapse • Kegel exercises → reduce stress incontinence from prolapse
Perineal body	• Located on pelvic floor • Fibromuscular tissue between vagina and rectum	• Transected in episiotomies
Pudendal nerve	• Originates from S2-S4 • Innervates structures of pelvic floor	• Perineal nerve block is directed toward this nerve

Table 3.5.3 - Pelvic floor structures

II. Cystocele

A. Pelvic organ prolapse can cause a dysfunctional urethral sphincter. This occurs if the loss of supporting structures allows the bladder to protrude posteriorly into the vaginal wall. This can lead to stress incontinence.

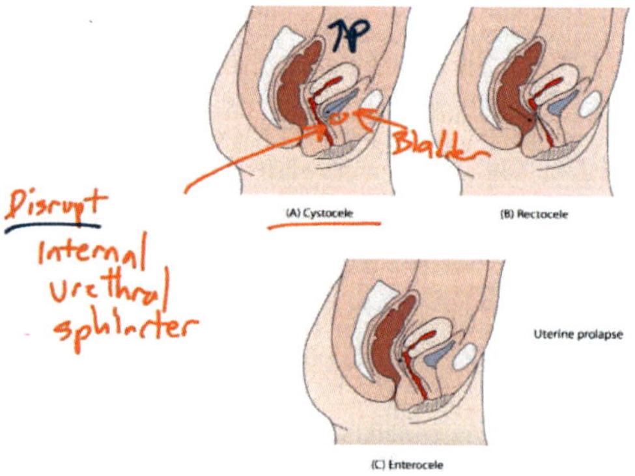

III. Rectocele

A. Loss of supporting structures can allow the rectum to protrude anteriorly into the vaginal wall. This can disrupt the anal sphincter (rare) or block the opening (common).

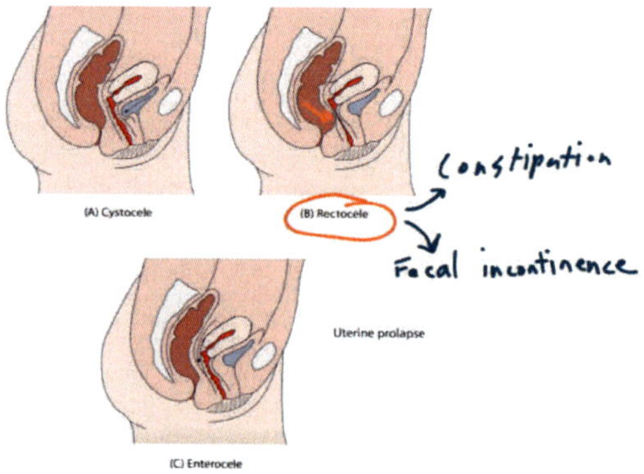

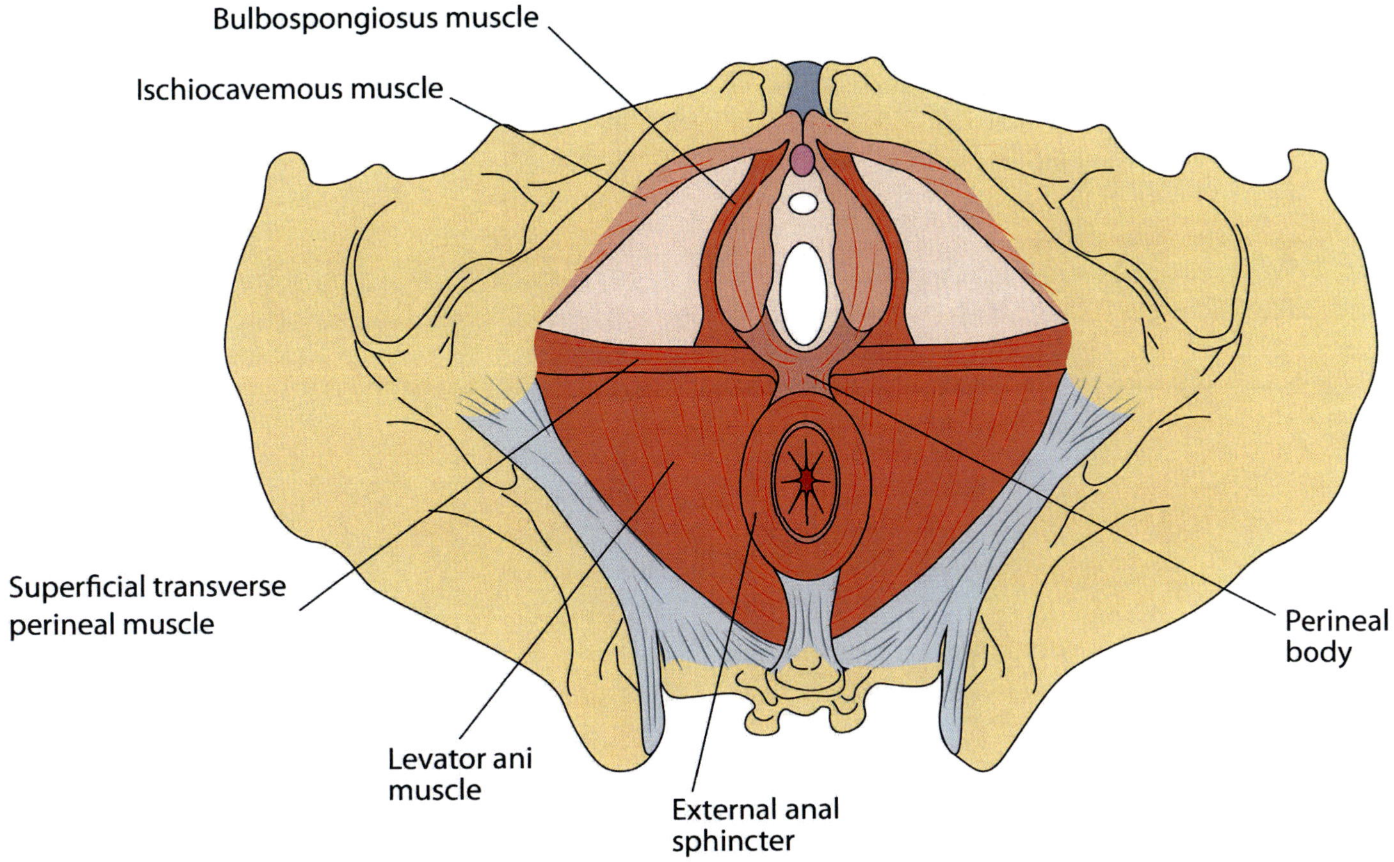

Figure 3.5.5 - Inferior view of the pelvic floor

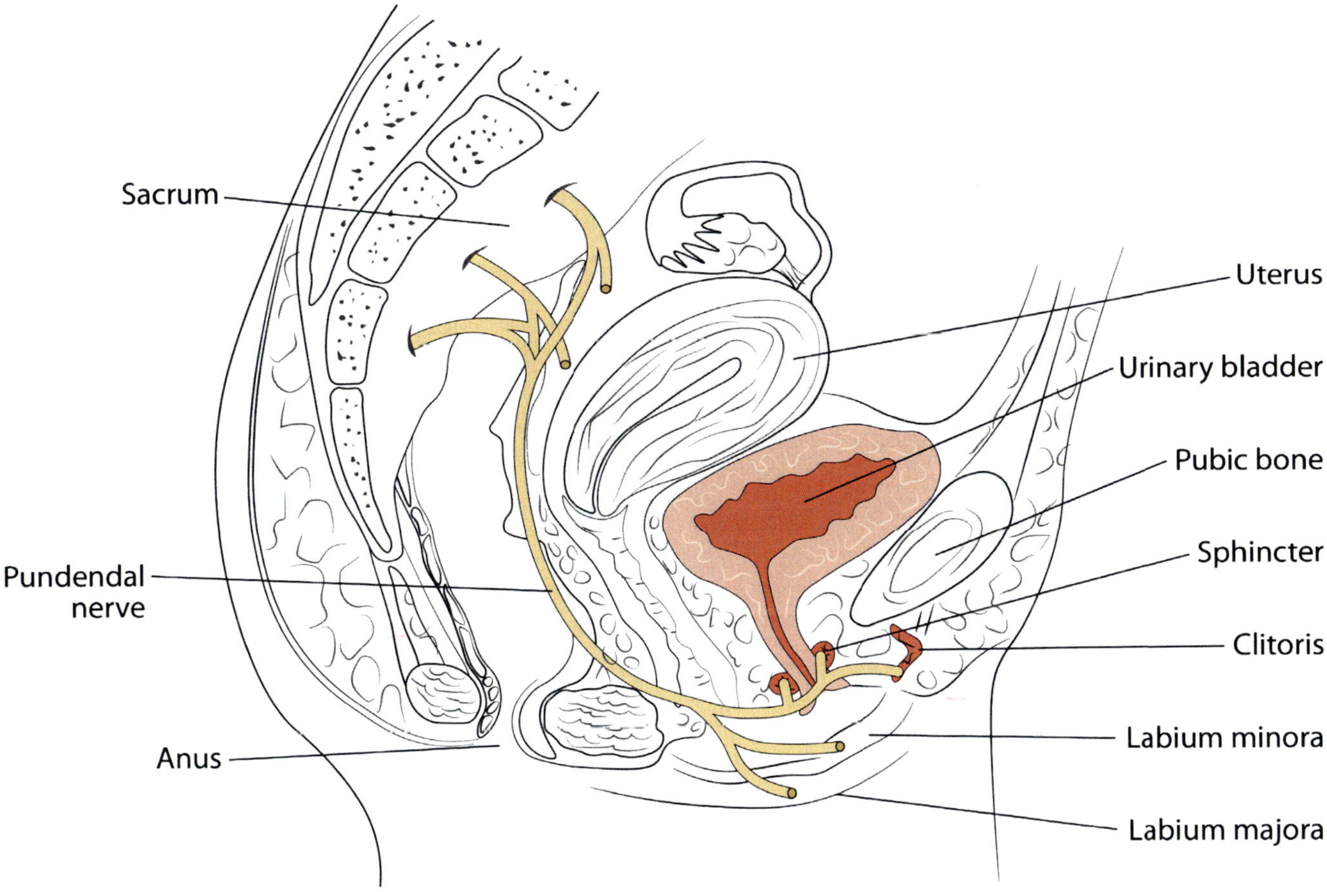

Figure 3.5.6 - Pudendal nerve

REVIEW QUESTIONS ?

1. A 78-year-old female has been experiencing unintentional loss of stool. She is diagnosed with pelvic organ prolapse. Is the anterior or posterior wall of the vaginal canal more likely to collapse inward during the Valsalva maneuver? What sphincter is most likely dysfunctional?

↑ Abdominal pressure → sphincter disruption
Urethral   Anal

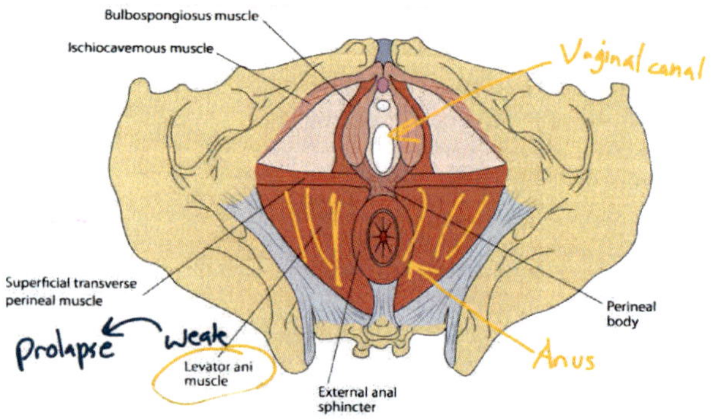

- **Answer: In the context of pelvic organ prolapse, increased abdominal pressure can disrupt important sphincters: the urethral sphincter and the anal sphincter. Fecal incontinence indicates rectocele and anal sphincter dysfunction → rectum pressures anteriorly into the vaginal wall.**

2. A 35-year-old pregnant female at 37 weeks' gestation presents to the hospital with spontaneous labor. The physician is concerned the vaginal opening is stretching and tearing to a degree that warrants an episiotomy. The episiotomy is performed, but continued stretching during labor causes tissue damage posteriorly. What anatomical structure(s) may be torn as a result of the tear?

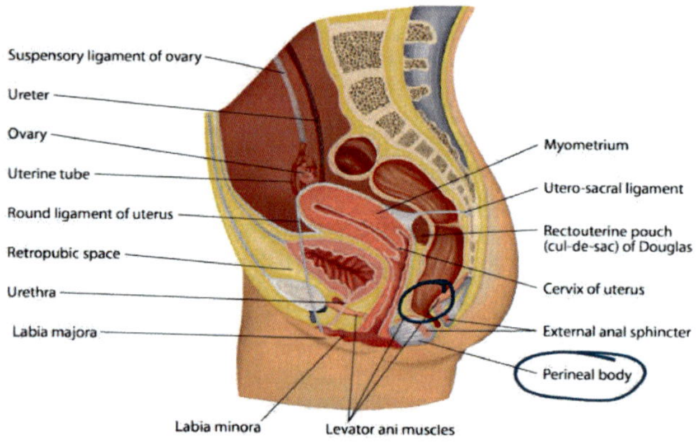

- **Answer: The perineal body is transected in an episiotomy. If the transected tissue extends too far posteriorly, the anal sphincter and the rectum can be damaged.**

Section IV - Male Reproductive Organs

Structure	Clinical Notes
Urethra	• Straddle injury → Injury to the anterior (bulbar) urethra → blood in scrotum • Pelvic fracture → Injury to the posterior (membranous) urethra → blood in retropubic space → prostate pushed superiorly and feel boggy
Prostate	• Prostatic hyperplasia (BPH) → urinary symptoms likely (close to urethra) • Prostate cancer → urinary symptoms possible if large enough, back pain (metastases via vertebral venous plexus)
Testicles	• Testicular torsion: Testicle wrapping around spermatic cord • Lymph drains to para-aortic nodes
Scrotum	• Varicocele: Dilated pampiniform plexus ("bag of worms" in scrotum) → does not transilluminate (light not easily seen through blood) • Hydrocele: Fluid in patent processus vaginalis → does transilluminate (light easily seen through serous fluid) • Lymph drains to superficial inguinal nodes

Table 3.5.4 - Important male structures

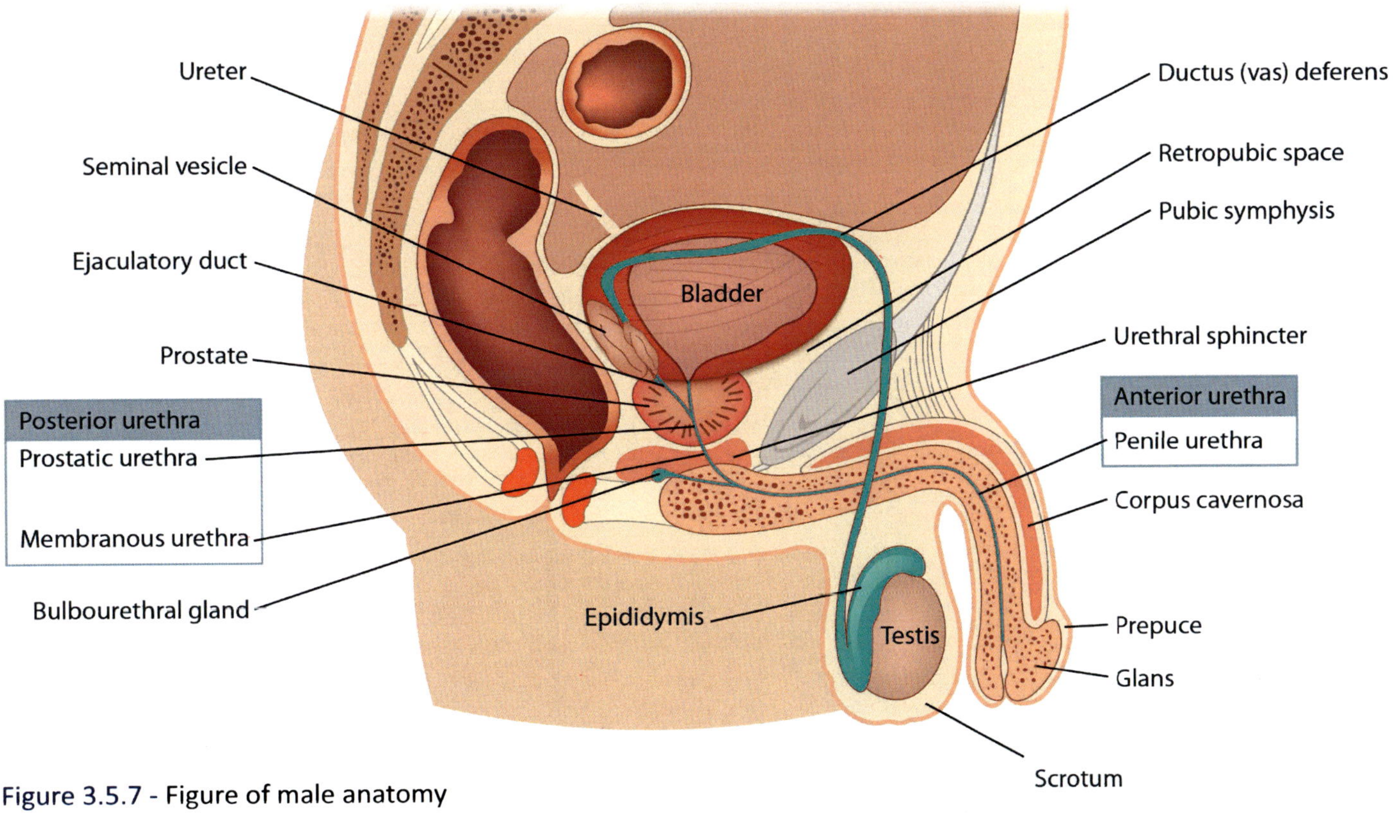

Figure 3.5.7 - Figure of male anatomy

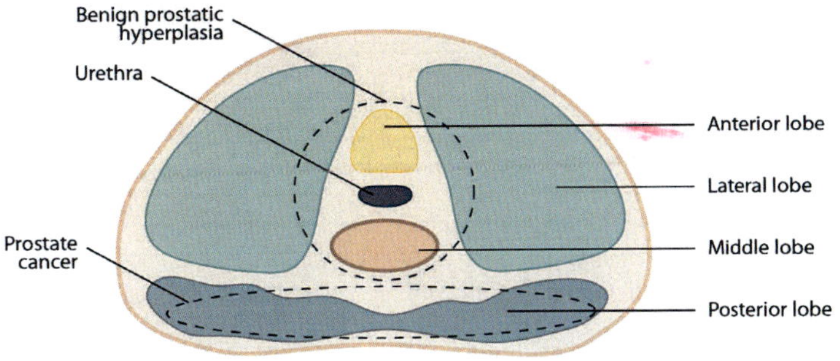

Figure 3.5.8 - Figure of prostate anatomy

II. Prostate Cancer Metastasis

A. Metastases from prostate cancer can reach the vertebral bodies using the vertebral venous plexus.

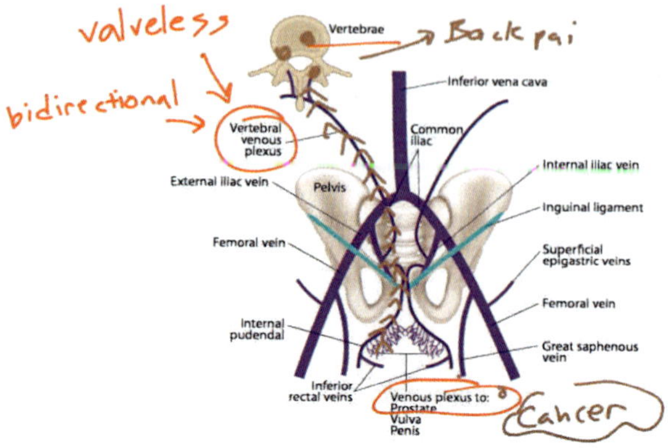

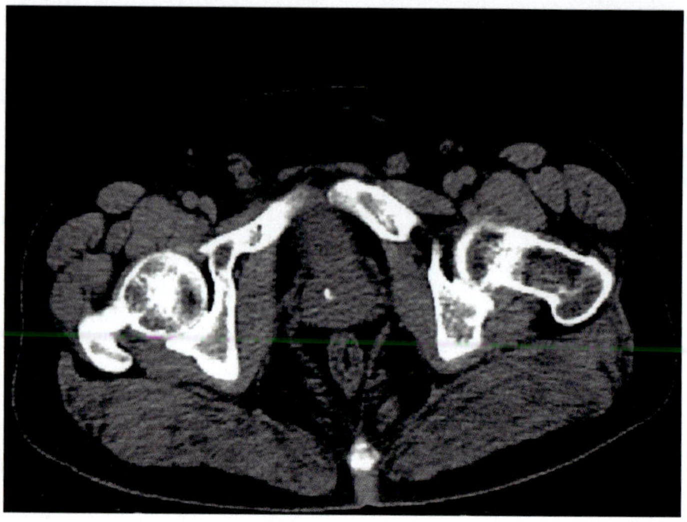

Figure 3.5.9 - Axial CT of Prostate Anatomy

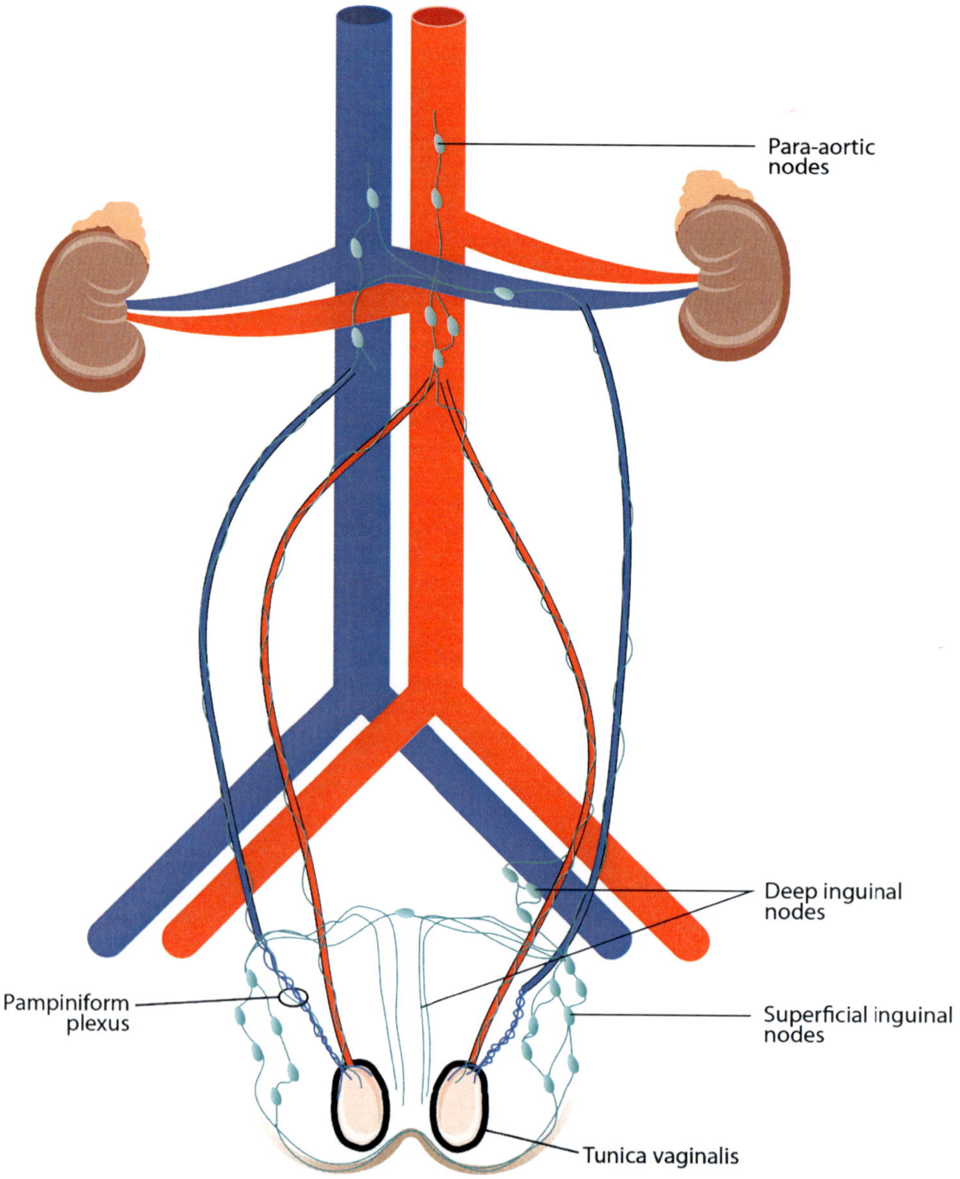

Figure 3.5.10 - Male lymphatic drainage

III. Identifying the Prostate on Imaging

A. The prostate is anterior to the anal canal.

B. The prostate may be seen posterior to the bladder if the inferior and anterior most part of the bladder dips protrudes forward.

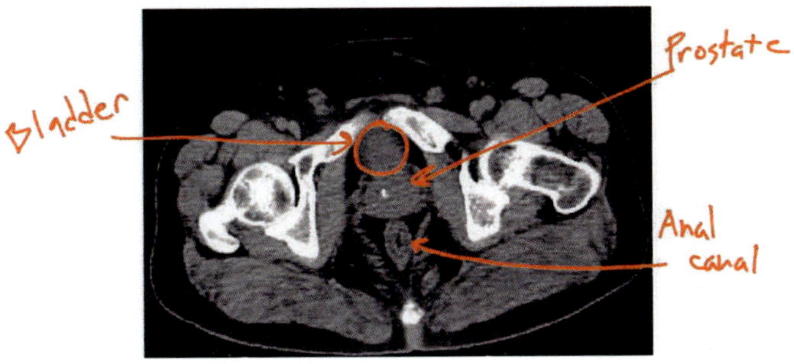

IV. Testicular Torsion

A. Occurs when the testicular artery and vein twist around the spermatic cord.

B. Can cause ischemia of the testis

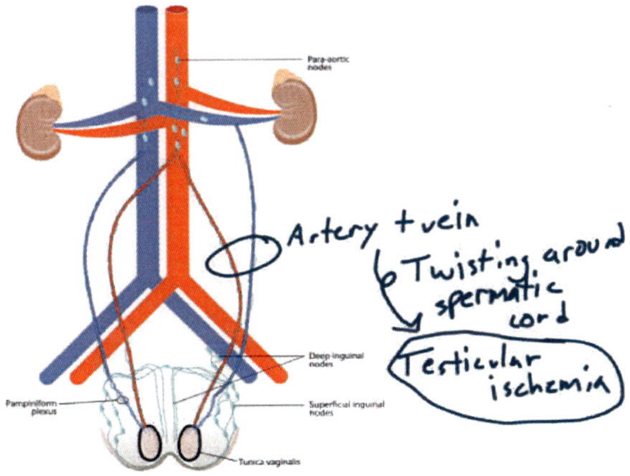

V. Hydrocele and Varicocele

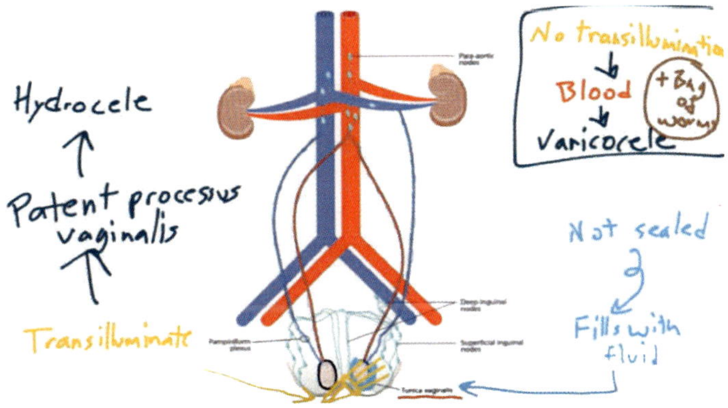

REVIEW QUESTIONS

1. A 6-year-old boy is brought to the emergency department following a playground accident. His mother states she didn't see what happened, but saw the boy crying on the ground near some tall playground equipment. On physical exam, the penis appears swollen and the scrotum appears fluid-filled throughout. The physician suspects a urethral injury. Assuming the physician is correct, is a pelvic fracture or a straddle injury more likely?

   - **Answer: A straddle injury is more likely. Pelvic fractures typically occur with high speed motor vehicle accidents. Furthermore, the scrotum filled with blood implicates an anterior straddle injury.**

2. A 33-year-old male is referred to an oncologist for possible testicular cancer. On physical exam, the oncologist palpates a genital mass as well as nearby palpable nodes. The superficial inguinal nodes on the patient's left side are tender and swollen. What does the physical exam indicate with regards to possible testicular cancer?

   - **Answer: Tender nodes often imply an infectious, rather than a cancerous etiology. This makes testicular cancer less likely. Additionally, the superficial inguinal nodes receive lymph from the scrotum, not the testicles. An infection of the scrotum is likely the cause of this patient's presentation.**

NEUROANATOMY

Section I - Neuroanatomy Overview

I. Neuroanatomy and Neuro-physiology are intricately connected. You cannot learn neuroanatomy in a meaningful way outside the context of the physiological functions of the relevant structures. See the Neurology Physiology chapter.

MUSCULOSKELETAL ANATOMY

Section I - Upper Trunk, Axillary, Musculocutaneous, Suprascapular Nerves

I. The brachial plexus is composed of roots, trunks, divisions, cords and branches. For board examination purposes, attention should be focused on only the trunks and branches. (See Table 3.6.1 - Brachial plexus nerves (axillary, musculocutaneous, suprascapular))

Nerve	Motor	Sensation	Injury Location	Presentation
Axillary	• Deltoid → shoulder abduction (>15°)	• Shoulder	• Surgical neck of humerus • Anterior dislocation • Upper trunk damage	• Arm at side
Musculocutaneous	• Biceps brachii → elbow flexion and forearm supination	• Lateral forearm	• Upper trunk damage	• Elbow extended • Pronated
Suprascapular	• Supraspinatus → shoulder abduction (0°-15°) • Infraspinatus → external rotation (Infection)	• Shoulder (above axillary)	• Upper trunk damage	• Arm at side • Internally rotated
Upper trunk (C5-C6 roots)	• Deltoid (axillary) → shoulder abduction (15°-90°) • Supraspinatus (suprascapular) → shoulder abduction (0°-15°) • Infraspinatus → external rotation (Infection) • Biceps brachii → elbow flexion and supination	• Shoulder • Lateral forearm	• Traumatic neck-shoulder separation (fall or delivery)	• Elbow extended (biceps dysfunction) • Pronated (biceps dysfunction) • Arm at side (deltoid dysfunction) • Internally rotated (infraspinatus dysfunction) • "Up by the deli inn"

Table 3.6.1 - Brachial plexus nerves (axillary, musculocutaneous, suprascapular)

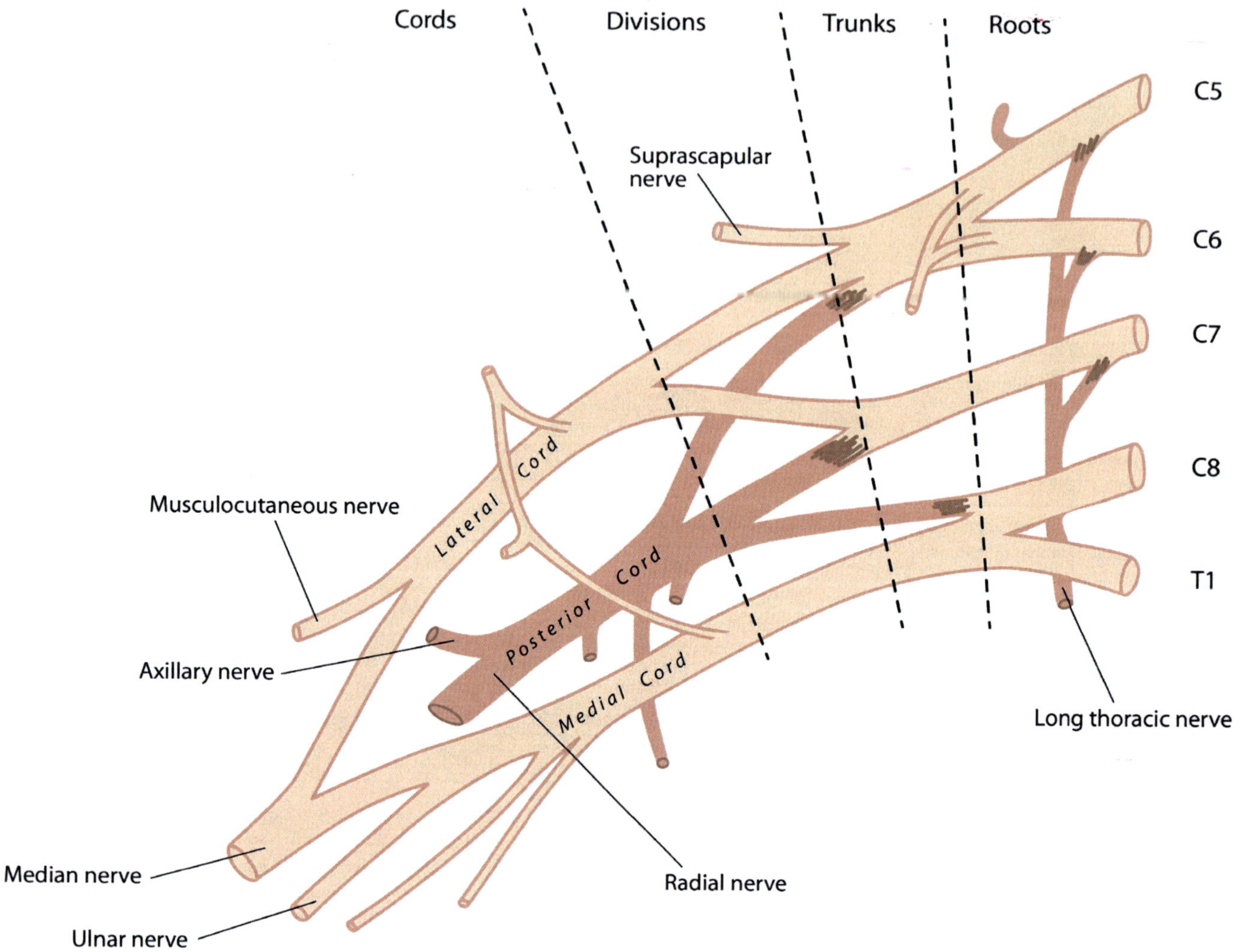

Figure 3.6.1 - Brachial plexus diagram

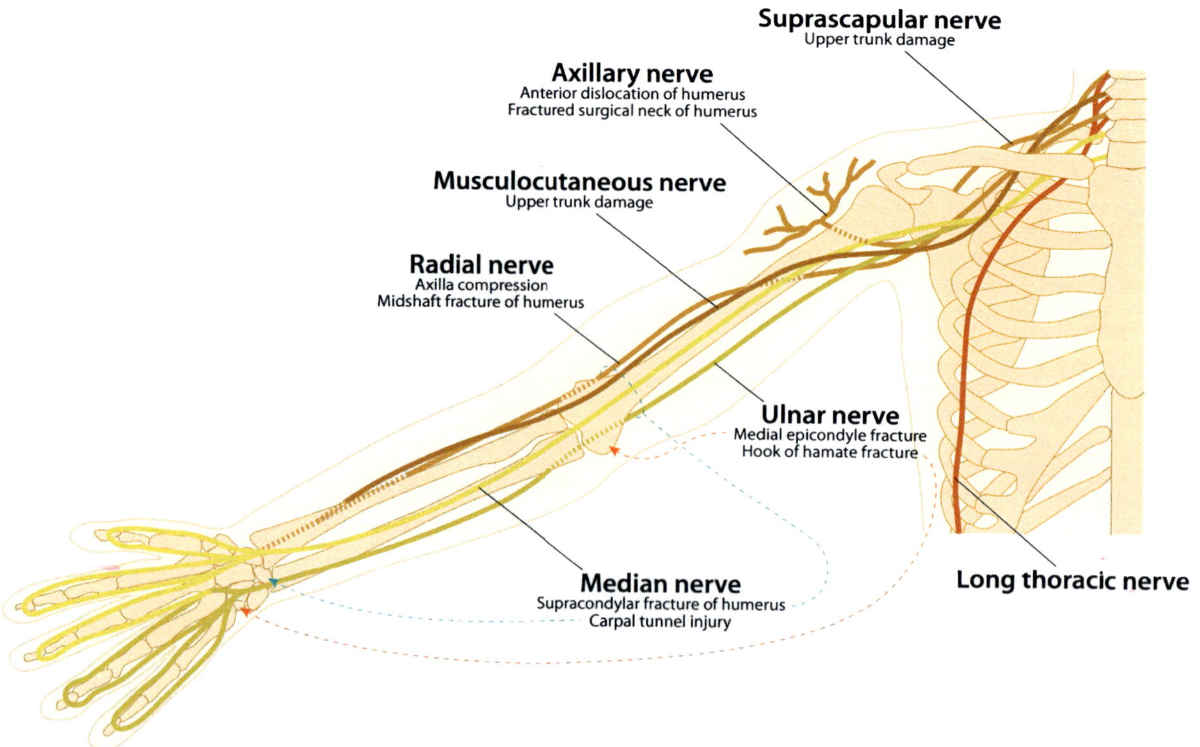

Figure 3.6.2 - Course of the brachial plexus nerves

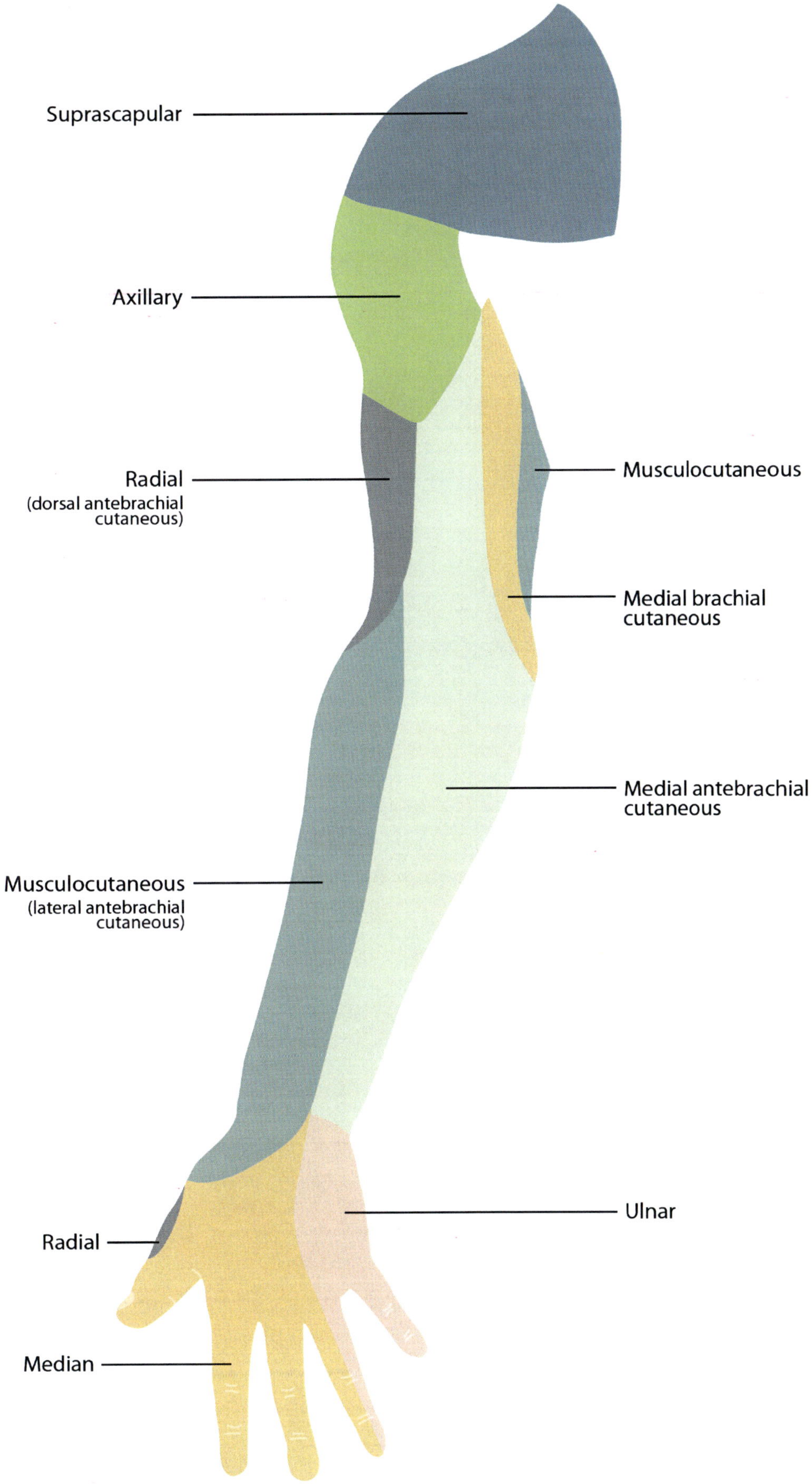

Figure 3.6.3 - Cutaneous innervation of the brachial plexus

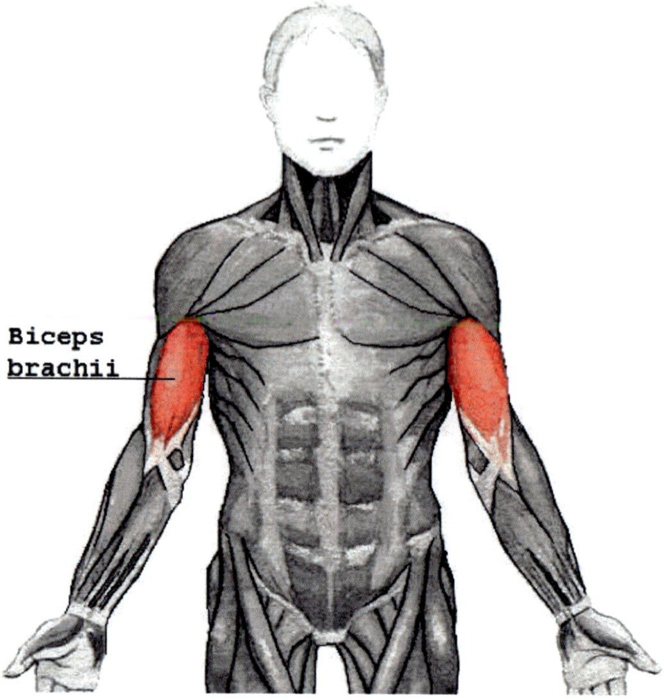

Figure 3.6.4 - Biceps brachii
By Bildbearbetning: sv:Användare:Chrizz (Transferred from sv.wikipedia to Commons.) [CC-BY-SA-3.0

A. Supination and Elbow Flexion

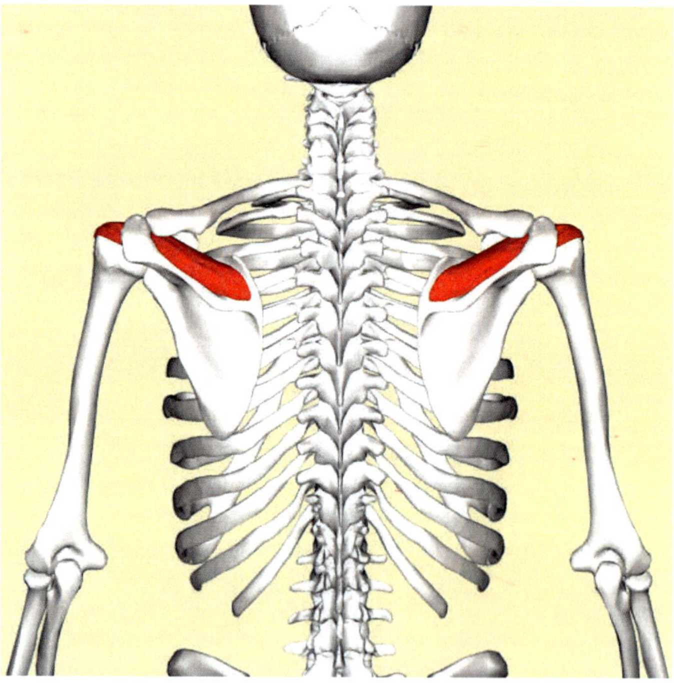

Figure 3.6.5 - Supination and elbow flexion
By Anatomography (en:Anatomography (setting page of this image)) [CC BY-SA 2.1 jp (https://creativecommons.org/licenses/by-sa/2.1/jp/deed.en)], via Wikimedia Commons

(http://creativecommons.org/licenses/by-sa/3.0/)], via Wikimedia Commons

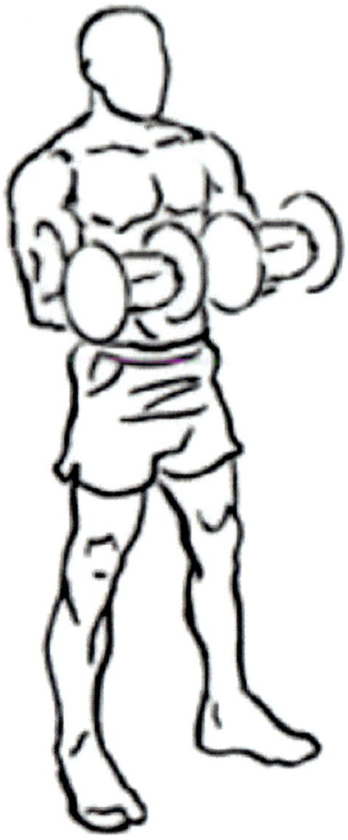

Figure 6.6 - Insert name
By Everkinetic (http://everkinetic.com/) [CC BY-SA 3.0 (https://creativecommons.org/licenses/by-sa/3.0)], via Wikimedia Commons

B. Suprascapular Muscle

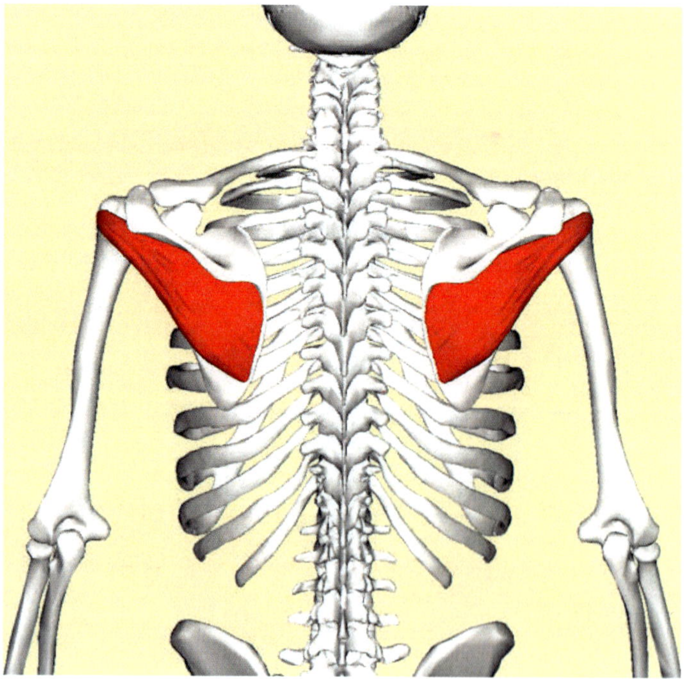

Figure 3.6.7 - Suprascapular muscle
By Anatomography (en:Anatomography (setting page of this image)) [CC BY-SA 2.1 jp (https://

creativecommons.org/licenses/by-sa/2.1/jp/deed.en)], via Wikimedia Commons

C. Infrascapular Muscle

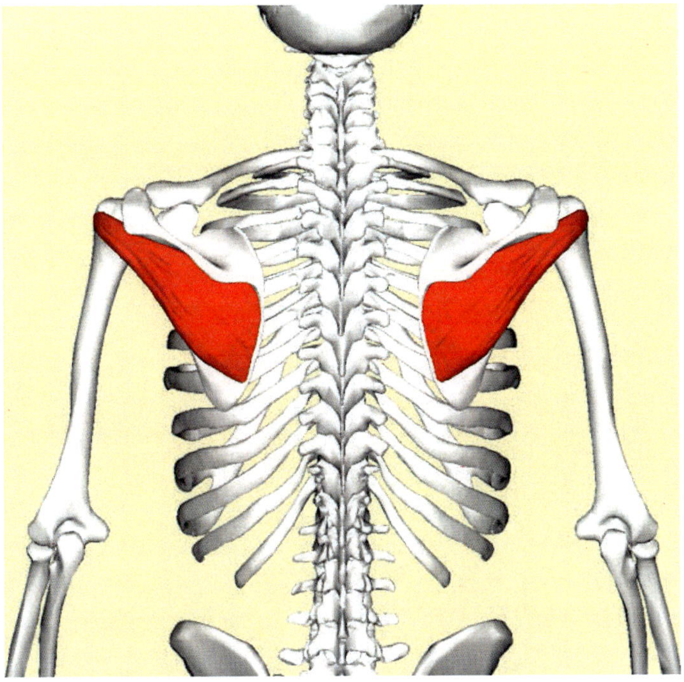

Figure 3.6.8 - Infrascapular muscle

By Anatomography (en:Anatomography (setting page of this image)) [CC BY-SA 2.1 jp (https://creativecommons.org/licenses/by-sa/2.1/jp/deed.en)], via Wikimedia Commons

II. Upper Trunk Damage

A. Forceful separation of the neck and shoulder can damage the upper trunk

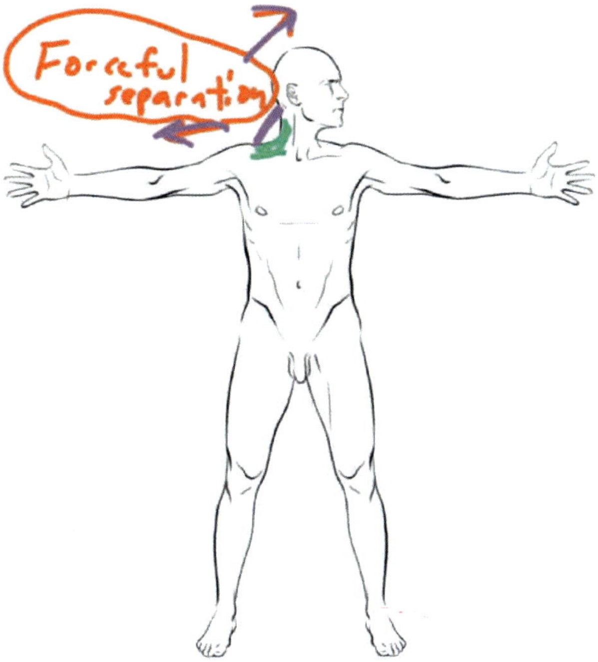

REVIEW QUESTIONS

1. A 45-year-old man presents to the emergency department holding his right shoulder and wincing in pain. His speech is incoherent and he appears intoxicated. A witness to the incident states the patient was hit multiple times in the arm with a pool cue. A radiograph of his arm is shown below. What neurological deficits will most likely be seen in this patient?

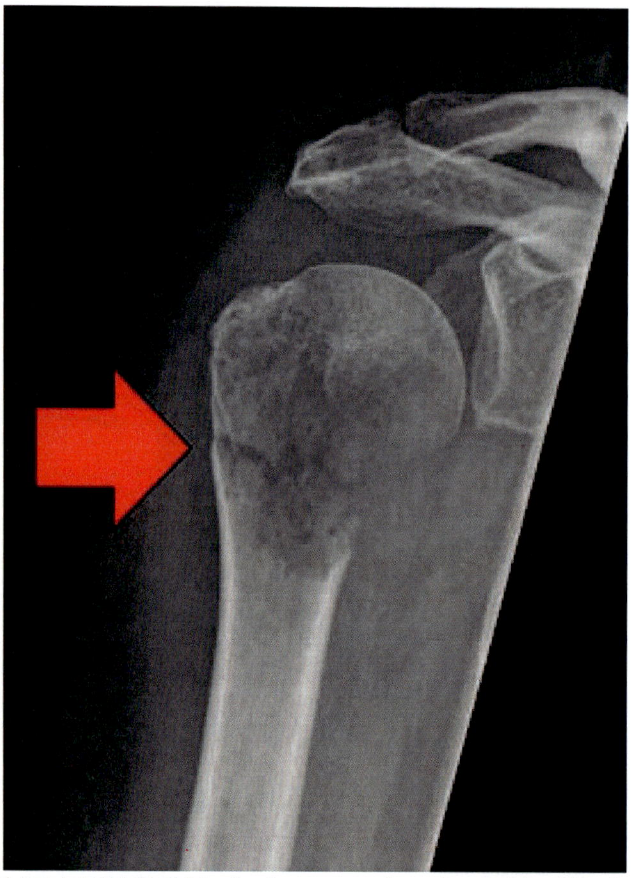

By Hellerhoff [CC BY-SA 3.0 (https://creativecommons.org/licenses/by-sa/3.0)], from Wikimedia Commons

- **Hopefully you can see on the image that the surgical neck of the humerus is broken.**
- **This should immediately make you think of the axillary nerve**
- **If this nerve is damaged, what muscle will be dysfunctional?**
  - **The deltoid, so the patient will be unable to abduct the shoulder**
- **What sensation will be lost?**
  - **Sensation over the deltoid**

2. A 14-year-old boy presents to a neurology clinic because his right arm "doesn't seem normal". He briefly states that he recently experienced some trauma. On exam, the patient cannot feel sensation in the region indicated by the physician's finger. Assuming the patient's presentation is the result of a denervated branch of the brachial plexus, what actions will the patient be unable to perform?

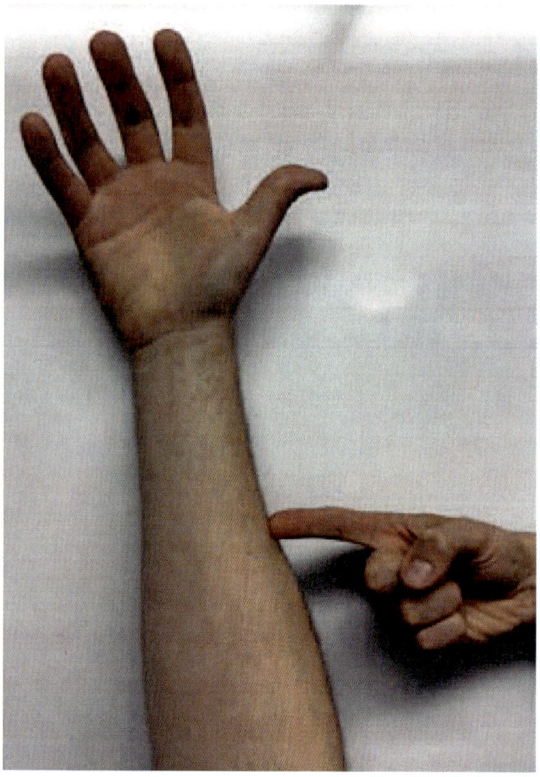

- **Answer: If a patient does not have sensation to this part of the arm, what branch of the brachial plexus should we think of?**
  - **Musculocutaneous nerve**
- **What muscle does the musculocutaneous nerve innervate?**
  - **Biceps brachii**
- **And what does that muscle do?**
  - **It allows flexion of the elbow joint and SUPINATION of the forearm**
- **So the patient would be unable to flex or supinate**

REVIEW QUESTIONS

3. A 23-year-old woman with cerebral palsy presents as a new patient to a family medicine clinic. The physician notices that her left arm is internally rotated. When asked if she can raise her arms to the ceiling, her right arm elevates but her left arm remains next to her body. Based only on these two physical exam findings, what muscles are not functioning?

- **Hopefully you noticed that this cerebral palsy patient has difficulty with external rotation. As you can see here, her arm is perpetually internally rotated.**
- **What muscle causes external rotation? (Remember the memory hook, infection)**
  - **Infraspinatus external rotation**
  - **So the left infraspinatus muscle is likely not functioning**
- **She also cannot raise her left arm, rather, she cannot abduct her left arm. What muscles abduct?**
  - **The supraspinatus abducts the first 15 degrees, the deltoid does the remainder**
- **So, she must have deficient supraspinatus and deltoid**

4. A 12-year-old girl presents to the emergency department following a traumatic fall from a tree she was climbing. Her parents state the impact forced her left ear to her left shoulder, creating a forceful stretch on the right side of her neck. Based on this history, the physician is concerned the patient may have damaged the upper trunk of her right brachial plexus. If the physician is correct, in what ways would the right arm be positioned?

- **If the upper trunk is damaged, what muscles are dysfunctional?**
  - **Recall the memory hook, up by the deli inn**
  - **Up for upper trunk**
  - **By for biceps**
  - **Deli for deltoid**
  - **Inn for infraspinatus**
- **If these muscles do not work, how would the right arm be positioned?**
  - **The biceps normally supinates and flexes, so her elbow would be extended and her forearm pronated**
  - **The deltoid normally abducts, so this patient's arm should be at her side**
  - **The infraspinatus normally externally rotates, so this patient's arm would likely be internally rotated**

Section II - Lower Trunk and the Median and Ulnar Nerves

Nerve	Motor	Sensation	Injury Location	Presentation
Median	• **Flexor digitorum profundus → flex wrist and PIP (2-3)** • **Lumbricals → flex MCP and extend PIP and DIP (2-3)** • Flexor digitorum superficialis → flex wrist and DIP • Pronator teres and quadratus → pronation • **Opponens pollicis → thumb opposition** • **Thenar eminence**	• Palmar: thenar and lateral 3.5 digits • Dorsal: lateral 3.5 digits	• Supracondylar fracture • Carpal tunnel	• Cannot make fist of digits 1-3 • Digits 2-3 frozen in resting hand position • Opponens pollicis fail → ape hand • Thenar atrophy
Ulnar	• **Flexor digitorum profundus → flexion of wrist and PIP (4-5)** • **Lumbricals → flex MCP and extend PIP and DIP (4-5)** • Dorsal interossei → abduct fingers • Palmar interossei → adduct fingers • **Hypothenar eminence**	• Palmar: medial 1.5 digits • Dorsal: medial 1.5 digits	• Medial epicondyle • Hook of hamate (Guyon's canal)	• Cannot make fist of digits 4 and 5 • Digits 4-5 frozen in resting hand position • Hypothenar atrophy
Lower trunk (C8-T1 roots)	• **Flexor digitorum profundus → flex wrist and PIP <u>(all digits)</u>** • **Lumbricals → flex MCP and extend PIP and DIP <u>(all digits)</u>**	• All digits	• Traumatic axilla stretching (falling and grabbing branch or delivery)	• <u>All digits</u> frozen in resting hand position • Numbness of medial 1.5 digits (ulnar loss)

Table 3.6.2 - Brachial plexus nerves (upper trunk, median, ulnar)

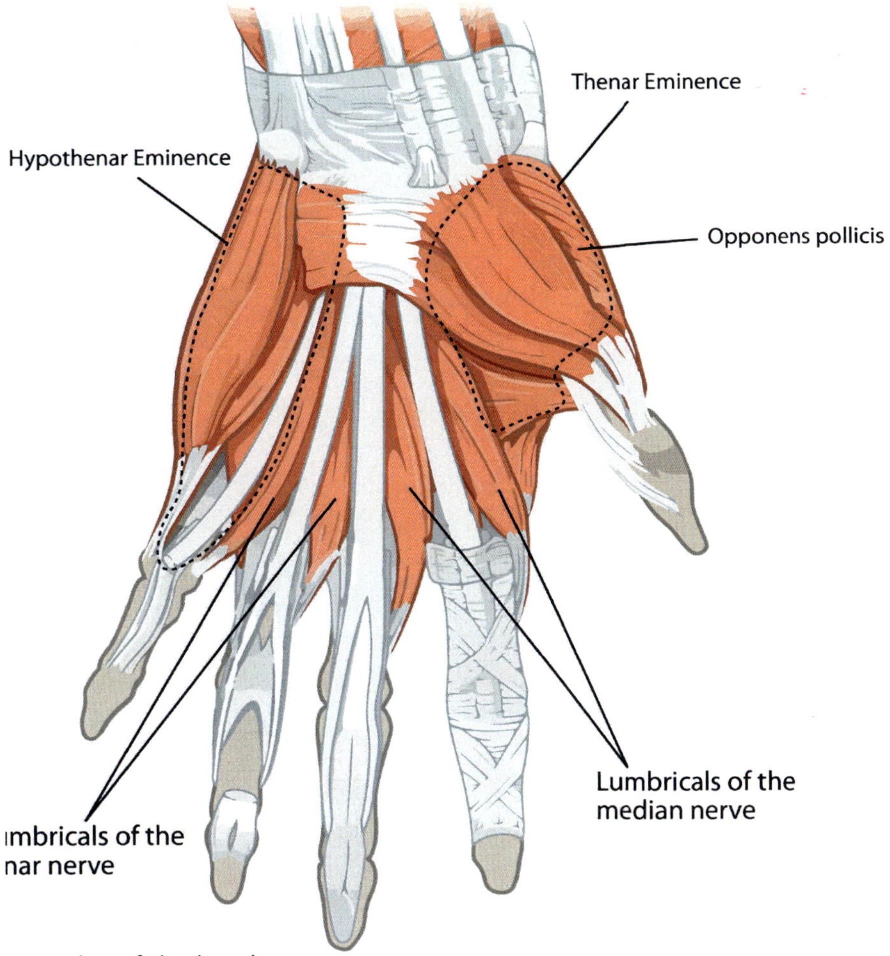

Figure 3.6.9 - Intrinsic muscles of the hand
By CFCF [CC BY-SA 4.0 (https:/creativecommons.org/licenses/by-sa/4.0)], from Wikimedia Commons, adjustments made

III. Opponens Pollicis Dysfunction

A. Without appropriate function of the opponens pollicis muscle, the patient will be unable to create a fist.

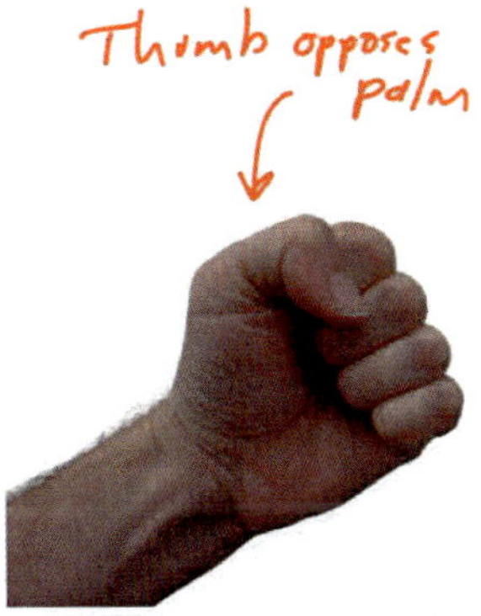

I. Ralpharama [GFDL (http://www.gnu.org/copyleft/fdl.html), CC-BY-SA-3.0 (http://creativecommons.org/licenses/by-sa/3.0/)], from Wikimedia Commons

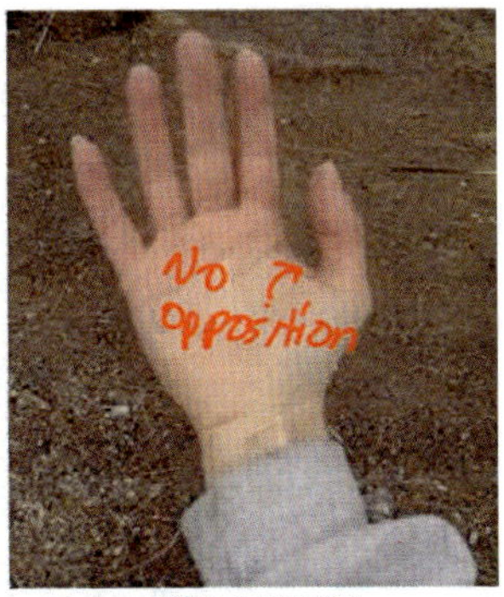

By Blurrybluesky [CC BY-SA 4.0 (https://creativecommons.org/licenses/by-sa/4.0)], from Wikimedia Commons

IV. Lumbrical Dysfunction

A. Without functional lumbricals, the patient will be unable to make a fist due to lost MCP flexion as well as PIP and DIP extension

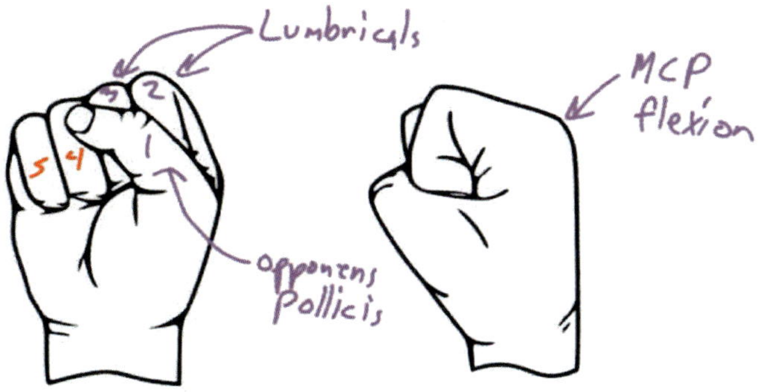

By Jean Paul GIBERT [CC BY 4.0 (https://creativecommons.org/licenses/by/4.0)], from Wikimedia Commons, adjustments made

V. Median Nerve Damage

A. Extending digits

1. Median nerve damage will result in lost lumbrical function. From resting hand position, digits 2 and 3 cannot extend the DIP and PIP joints.

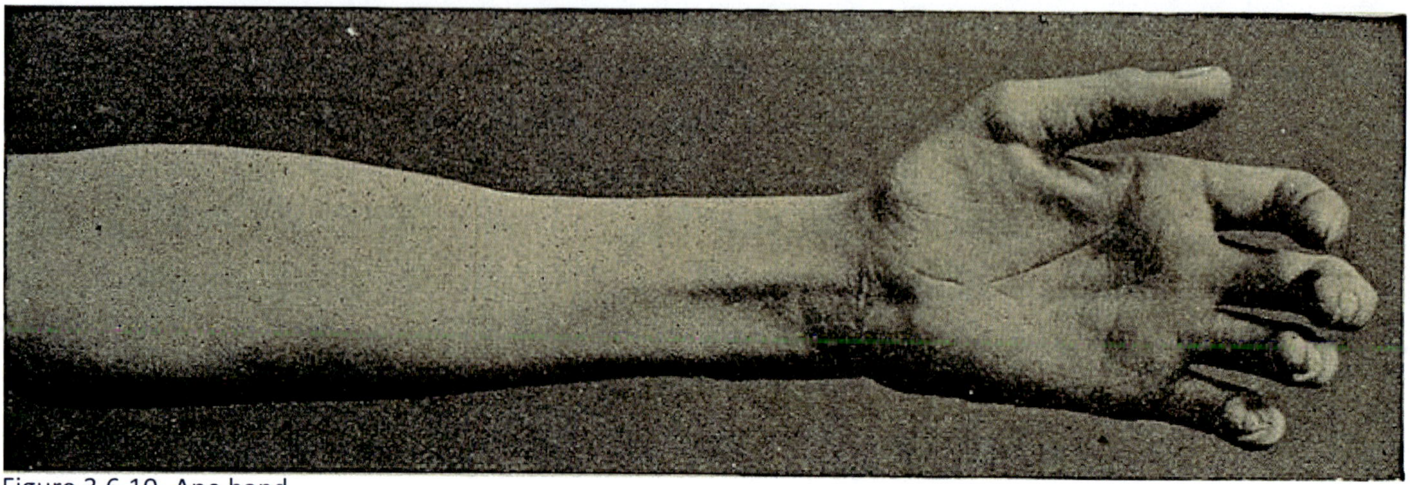

Figure 3.6.10- Ape hand
Public domain/Flickr

B. Flexing digits

1. Median nerve damage will result in lost lumbrical function in digits 2 and 3. This means the patient cannot make a fist with MCP dysfunction.
2. The flexor digitorum profundus will also be dysfunctional with median nerve damage. This results in lack of PIP flexion of digits 2 and 3.

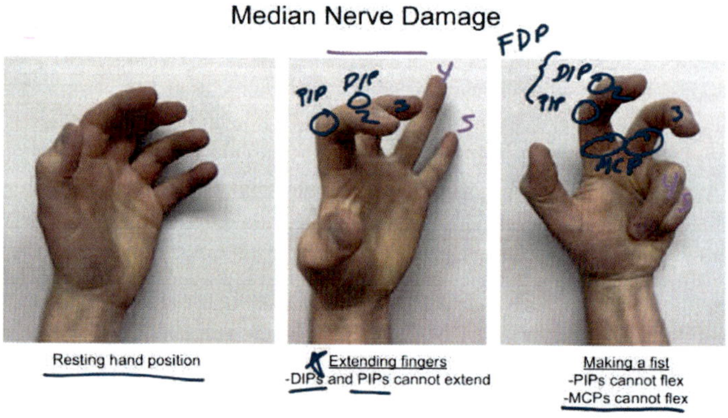

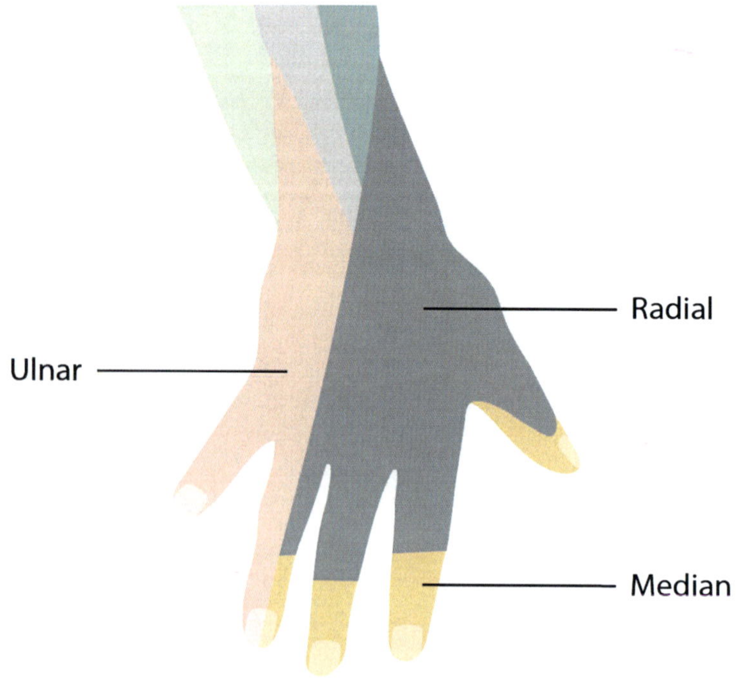

Figure 3.6.11 - Cutaneous Innervation of the Brachial Plexus (Dorsal Hand View)

VI. Ulnar Nerve Damage

A. Extending digits

1. Ulnar nerve damage results in loss of lumbrical function. With lumbrical dysfunction, the DIP and PIP joints of digits 4 and 5 will be unable to extend from resting hand position

B. Flexing digits

1. Median nerve damage will result in lost lumbrical function in digits 4 and 5. This means the patient cannot make a fist with MCP dysfunction.

2. The flexor digitorum profundus will also be dysfunctional with median nerve damage. This results in lack of PIP flexion of digits 4 and 5.

Ulnar Nerve Damage

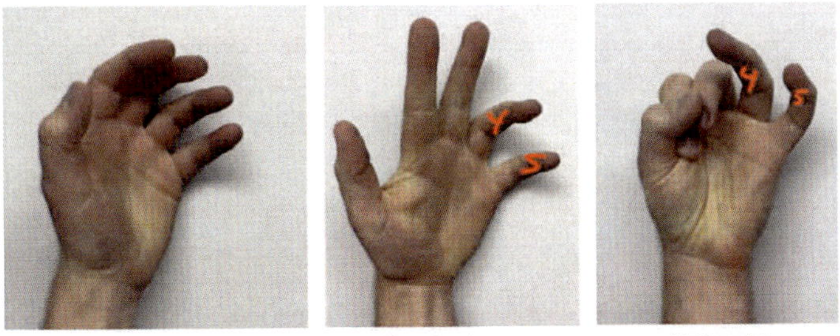

Resting hand position

Extending fingers
-DIPs and PIPs cannot extend

Making a fist
-PIPs cannot flex
-MCPs cannot flex

VII. Lower Trunk Damage

A. The lower trunk can be damaged with stretching or prolonged compression of the axilla.

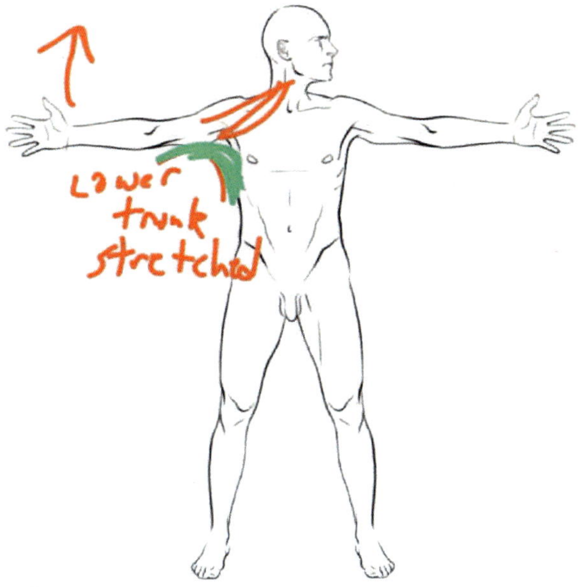

REVIEW QUESTIONS ?

1. A 14-year-old male presents to the emergency department following a motor vehicle accident. He was the unrestrained passenger when a truck collided with the passenger door at high speed. The boy is alert and oriented, but is crying in pain while holding is left arm. A radiograph is obtained which is shown below. Based on the radiographic findings, the physician suspects damage to a nerve. Based on these findings how would the patient's hand most likely appear if asked to make a fist?

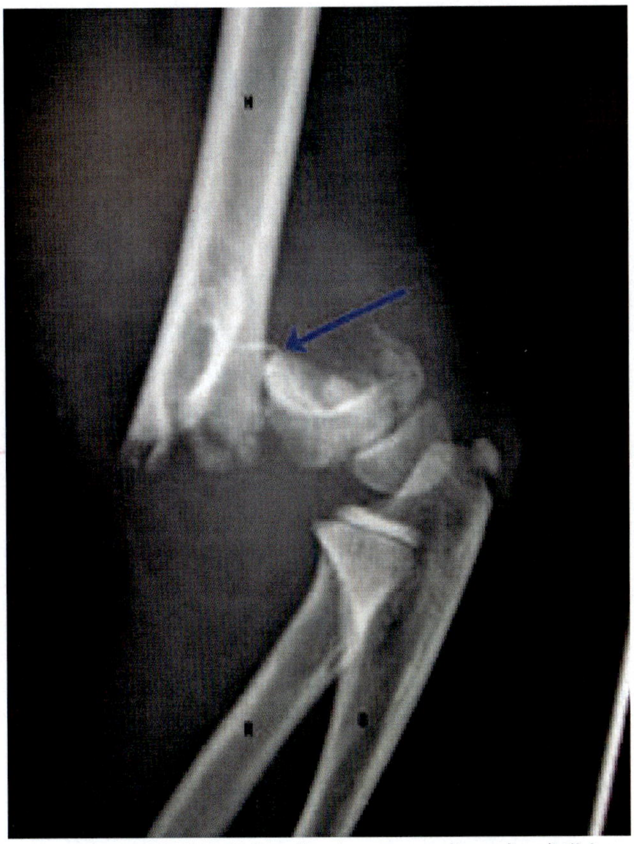

By James Heilman, MD [CC BY-SA 3.0 (https://creativecommons.org/licenses/by-sa/3.0)], from Wikimedia Commons

- **Answer: The median nerve is adjacent to the humerus at the supracondylar area. Supracondylar fracture could lesion the median nerve which is assumed in this patient. When asked to make a fist, the patient will be unable to flex digits 2 and 3 into a fist.**

REVIEW QUESTIONS

2. A 46-year-old man trips and falls on his left outstretched hand. His left hand is extremely painful. An urgent care physician orders a radiograph which reveals a fracture in his hand. The man is asked to extend all of the digits of his left hand and then a picture is taken which is shown below. What part of his hand is most likely fractured? What sensation is most likely lost?

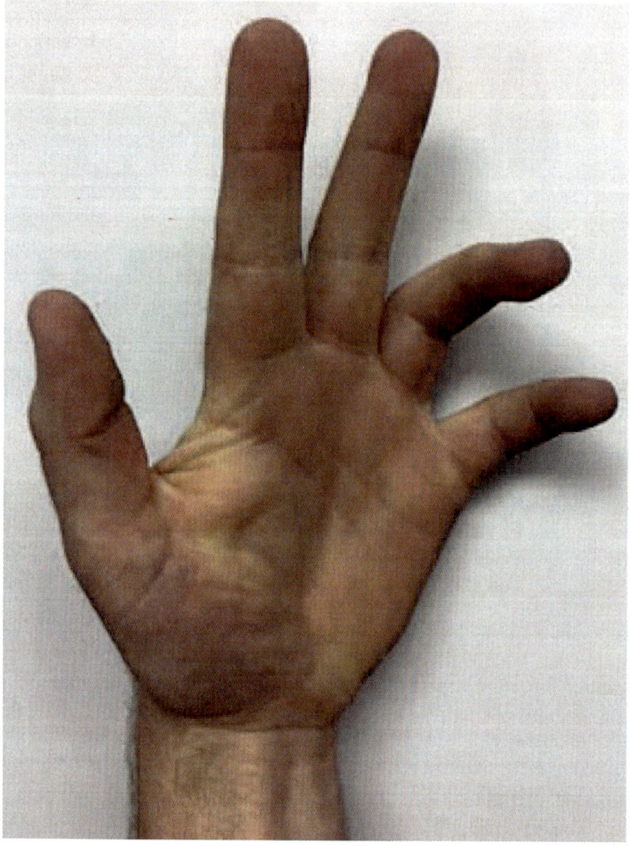

- **Answer: The patient is unable to extend digits 4 and 5. This indicates dysfunction of the lumbricals innervated by the ulnar nerve. The ulnar nerve can be damaged at the medial epicondyle or the hook of the hamate. With a fall on an outstretched hand, damage to the hamate is more likely.**
- **Sensation will be diminished on the palmar and dorsal surface of the medial 1.5 digits.**

3. A 16-year-old boy is brought to the emergency department by his parents after he fell out of a tree. After free falling for 2 seconds, he grabbed a branch with his right hand. The rest of his body continued falling until his fall was abruptly stopped when grabbing this branch. Almost immediately, the boy let go of the branch and fell the rest of the way to the ground. He is crying in pain but does not localize it. Based on the scenario, the physician is concerned about damage to the brachial plexus. If damage to the brachial plexus occurred, name two muscle groups which may be denervated?

- **Answer: Forceful stretching of the axilla can damage the lower trunk. The muscle groups most likely to result in physical exam findings if dysfunctional are the lumbricals and the flexor digitorum profundus.**
  - **With suspected lower trunk lesions, the muscles innervated by both the median and ulnar nerves should be considered (i.e. digits 2 through 5).**

Section III - Radial and Long Thoracic Nerves

Nerve	Motor	Sensation	Injury Location	Presentation
Radial	• Triceps → elbow extension • Extensor carpi radialis → wrist extension • Extensor carpi ulnaris → wrist adduction • Extensor digitorum → finger extension (digits 2-5)	• Dorsal: thumb and lateral portion of hand • Lateral upper arm	• Axilla compression • Mid-shaft fractures	• Elbow flexed (unless mid-shaft fracture) • Wrist drop
Long thoracic	• Serratus anterior → anchor scapula to thorax	• NA	• Mastectomy • Stab wounds	• Winged scapula

Table 3.6.3 - Brachial plexus nerves (lower trunk, radial, long thoracic)

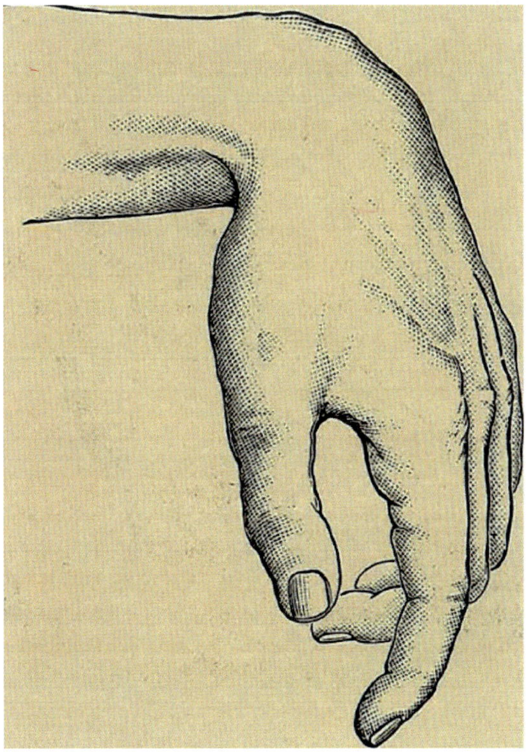

Figure 3.6.12 - Wrist Drop
Public domain/Flickr

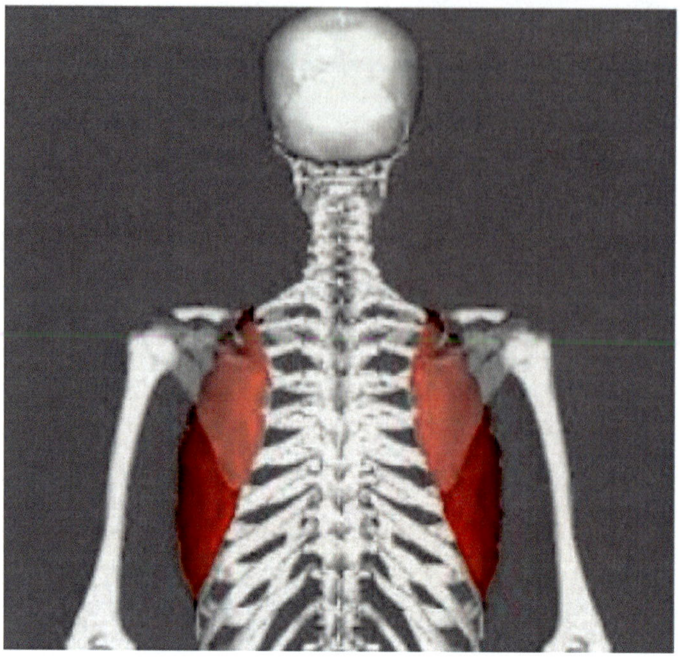

Figure 3.6.13 - Serratus Anterior (Posterior View)
By Anatomography (en:Anatomography (setting page of this image)) [CC BY-SA 2.1 jp (https://creativecommons.org/licenses/by-sa/2.1/jp/deed.en)], via Wikimedia Commons

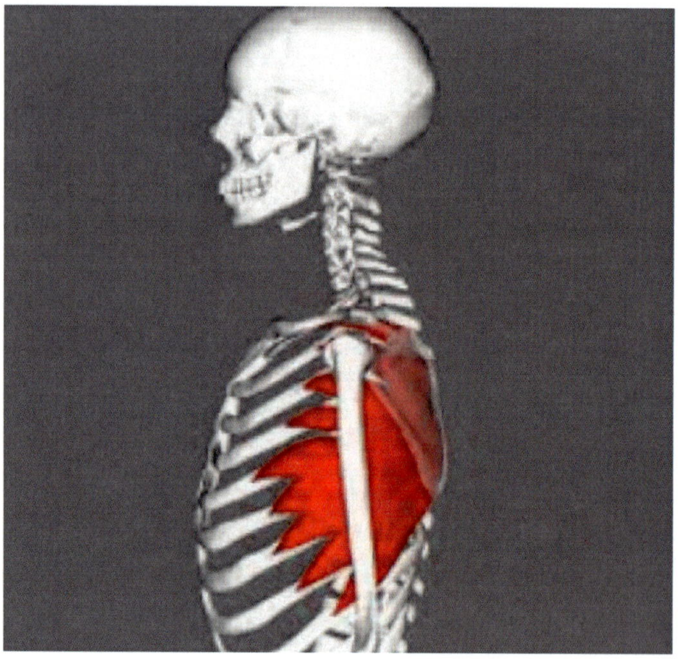

Figure 3.6.14 - Serratus Anterior (Lateral View)
By Anatomography (en:Anatomography (setting page of this image)) [CC BY-SA 2.1 jp (https://creativecommons.org/licenses/by-sa/2.1/jp/deed.en)], via Wikimedia Commons

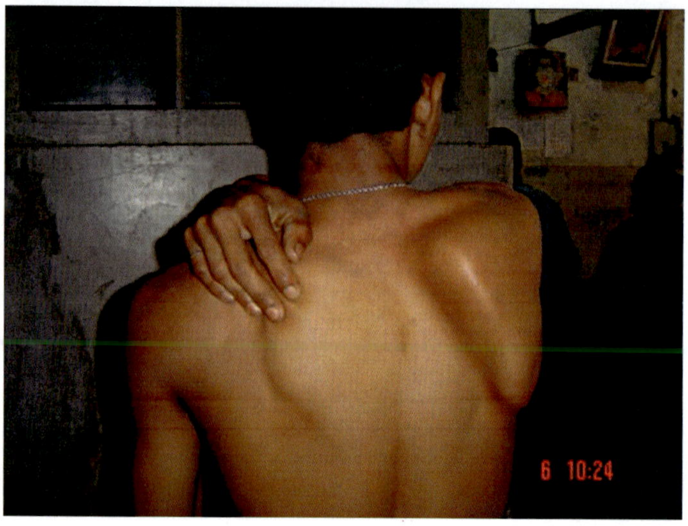

Figure 3.6.15 - Winged Scapula
Dwaipayanc at the English language Wikipedia [CC-BY-SA-3.0 (http://creativecommons.org/licenses/by-sa/3.0/)], from Wikimedia Commons

REVIEW QUESTIONS ?

1. A 23-year-old male wakes up after a long weekend of drinking alcohol. During this time the patient was also involved in bar fights and sustained many undiagnosed injuries. On physical examination, he cannot extend his right wrist or contract his right triceps muscle. Where in its course is the defective nerve most likely damaged?

   - **Answer: Loss of wrist and elbow extension indicates radial nerve damage. With loss of triceps function, a proximal lesion is more likely. Proximal lesions typically occur at the axilla.**
   - **A distal radial nerve lesion would spare triceps function. These lesions typically occur with mid-shaft fractures of the humerus.**

I. Thoracic outlet

A. Superior border: clavicle

B. Inferior border: first rib

C. Several structures traverse outlet

1. Subclavian artery
2. Subclavian vein
3. Brachial plexus

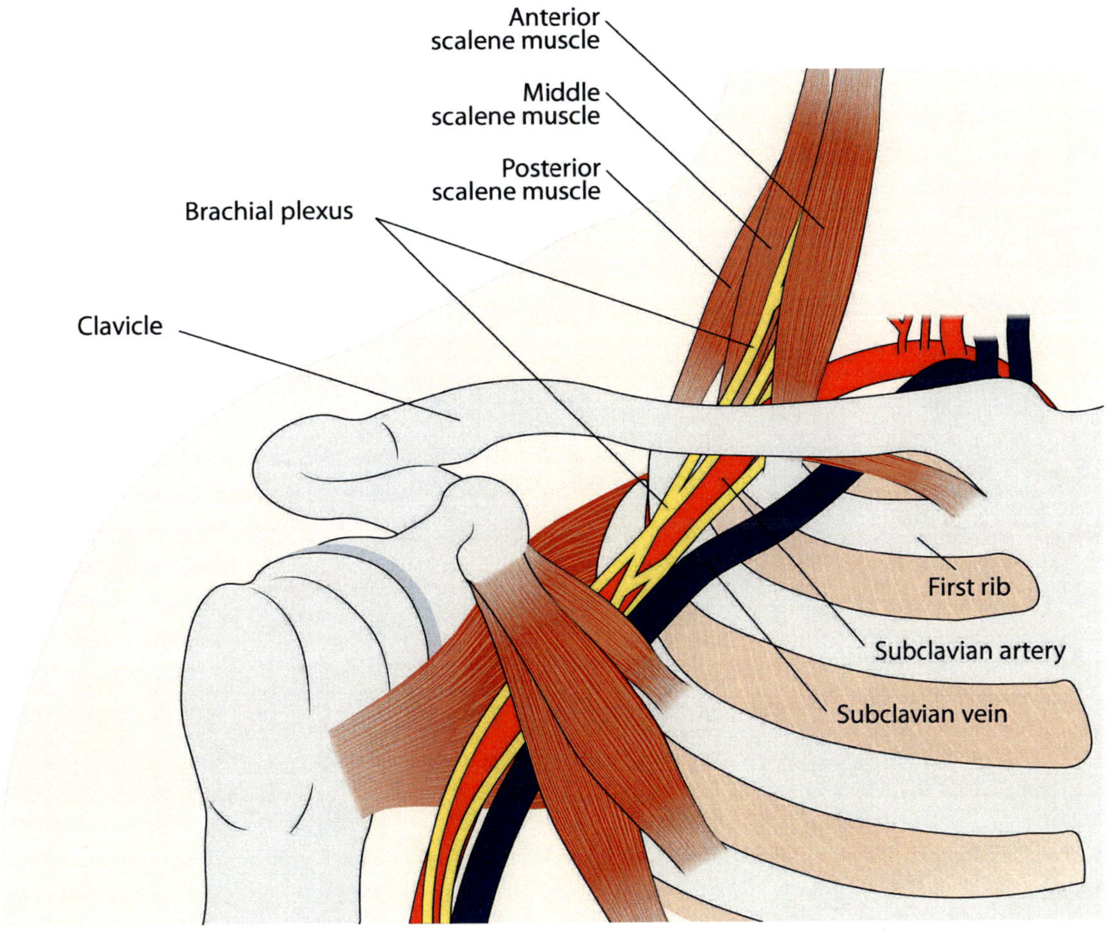

Figure 3.6.16 - Thoracic outlet

II. Thoracic outlet syndrome

A. Compression of certain components within the thoracic outlet leads to symptoms

1. Brachial plexus (lower trunk) → weakness, pain, tingling
2. Subclavian artery → exertional arm pain (claudication)
3. Subclavian vein → venous congestion (swelling)

III. Scalene triangle

A. Boundaries: anterior scalene, middle scalene and clavicle

B. Can cause thoracic outlet syndrome
  1. Overuse injury or inflammation of scalene muscles
  2. Anomalous cervical rib
C. Targeted in brachial plexus nerve block

IV. Rotator cuff
  A. Composed of four muscles
  B. Stabilizes the glenohumeral (shoulder) joint
  C. Understand function and recognize pathology

Rotator Cuff Muscle	Function	Innervation	Notes
Supraspinatus	Abduction (0°-15°)	Suprascapular nerve	Tendon impingement between acromion and humerus → pain with abduction Injury → weak abduction
Infraspinatus	External rotation	Suprascapular nerve	Nerve injury → weak external rotation "Infection"
Teres minor	External rotation Adduction	Axillary nerve	Nerve injury → weak external rotation
Subscapularis	Internal rotation Adduction	Upper subscapular nerve Lower subscapular nerve	Nerve injury → weak internal rotation "Sub-I"

Table 3.6.4 - Rotator cuff muscles

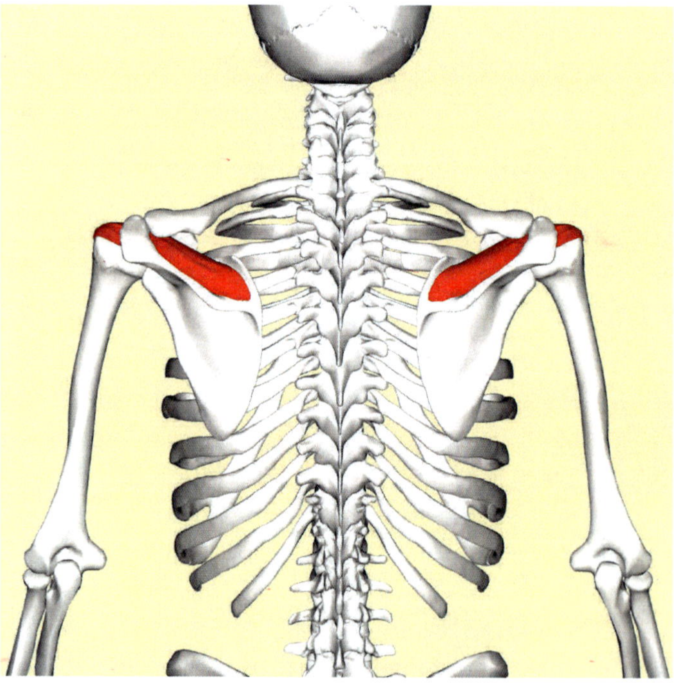

Figure 3.6.17 - Supraspinatus muscle
By Anatomography (en:Anatomography (setting page of this image)) [CC BY-SA 2.1 jp (https://creativecommons.org/licenses/by-sa/2.1/jp/deed.en)], via Wikimedia Commons

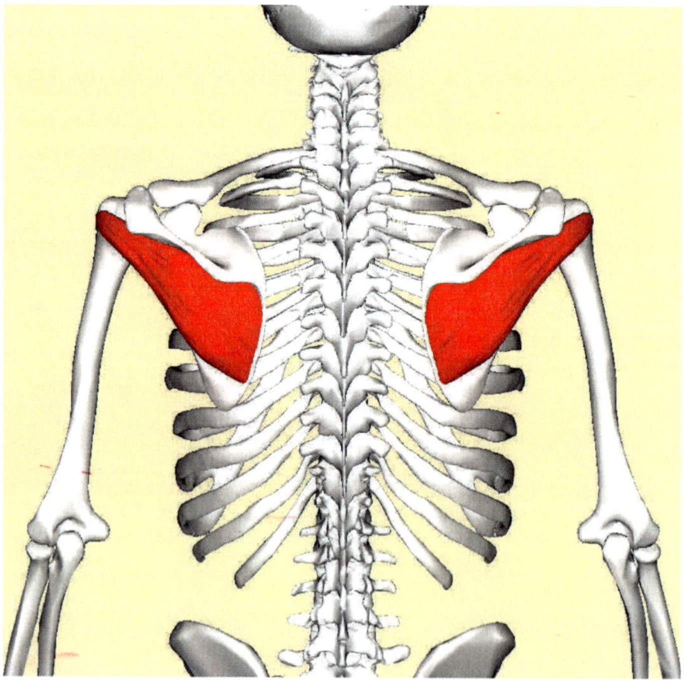

Figure 3.6.18 - Infraspinatus Muscle
By Anatomography (en:Anatomography (setting page of this image)) [CC BY-SA 2.1 jp (https://creativecommons.org/licenses/by-sa/2.1/jp/deed.en)], via Wikimedia Commons

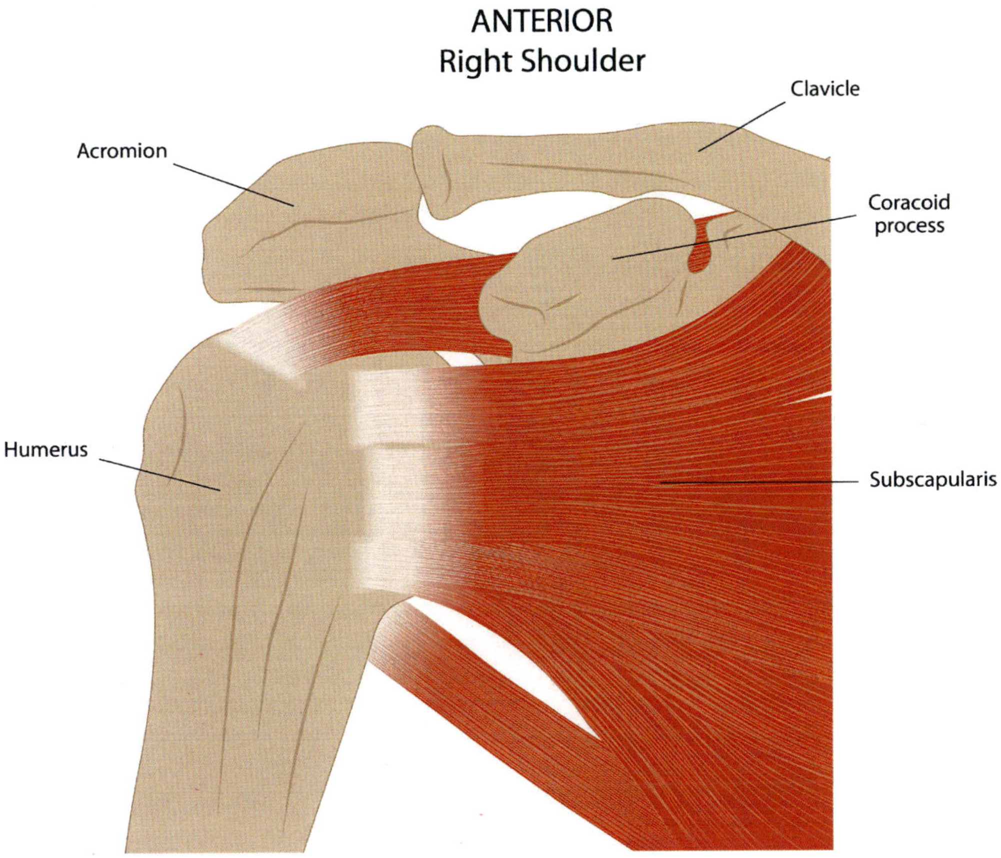

Figure 3.6.19 - Anterior shoulder

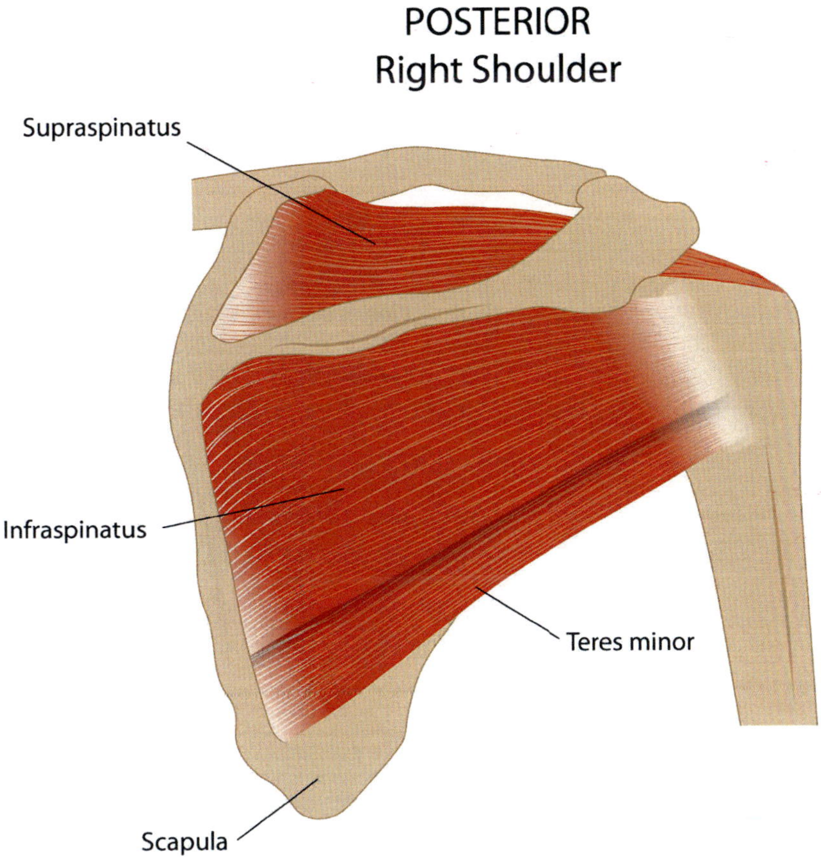

Figure 3.6.20 - Posterior shoulder

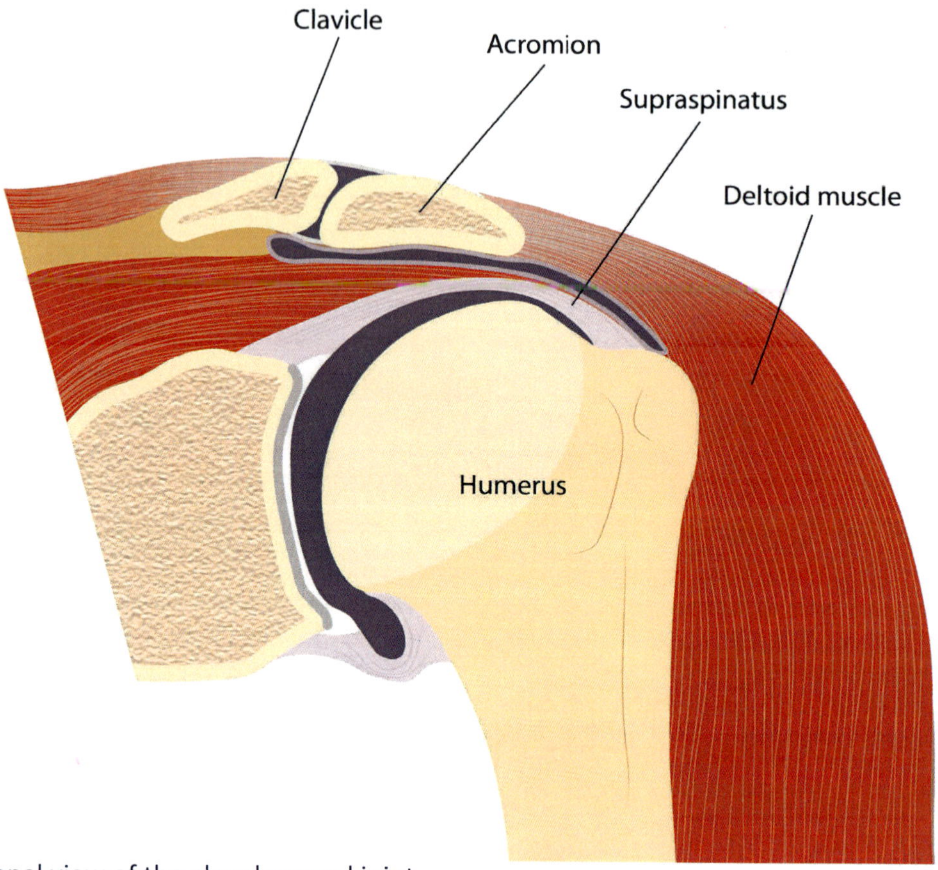

Figure 3.6.21 - Coronal view of the glenohumeral joint

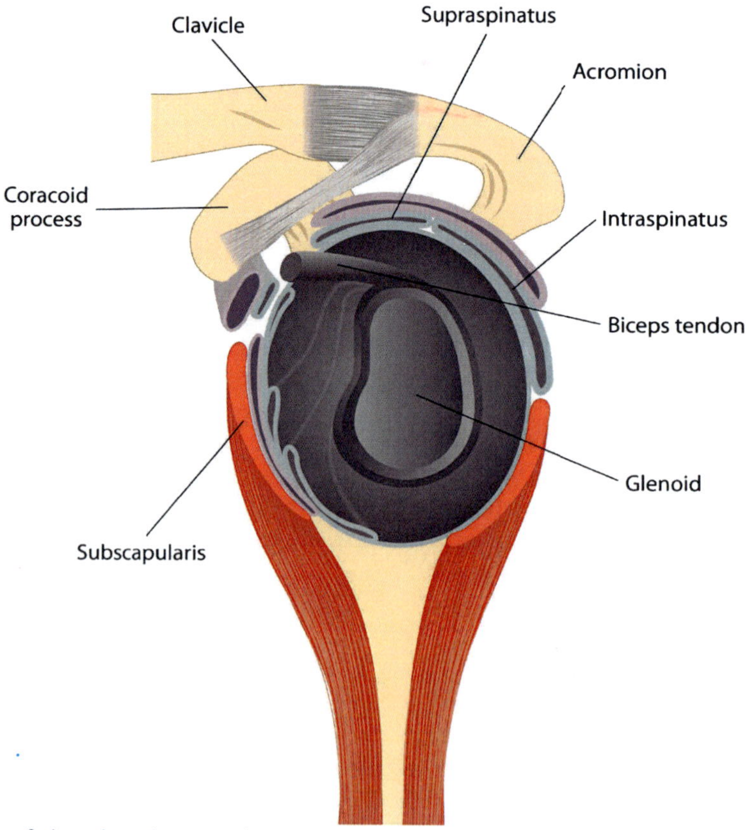

Figure 3.6.22 - Sagittal view of the glenohumeral joint

Muscle	Function	Innervation
Latissimus dorsi	Extension Adduction	Thoracodorsal nerve
Trapezius	Scapula movement	CN XI: Spinal accessory nerve
Sternocleidomastoid	Rotate neck Flex neck (bilateral contraction)	CN XI: Spinal accessory nerve
Pectoralis major	Shoulder flexion	Pectoral nerves

Table 3.6.5 - Important shoulder region muscles

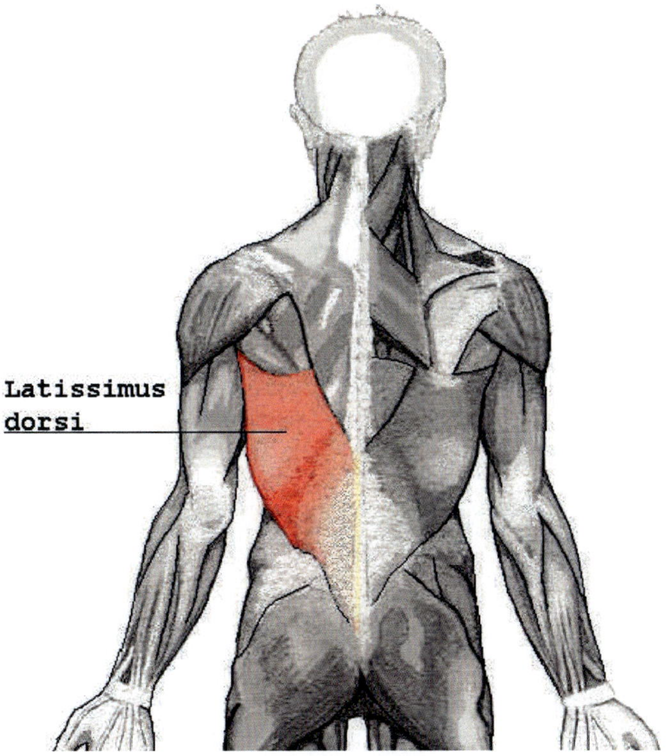

Figure 3.6.23 - Latissimus dorsi muscle

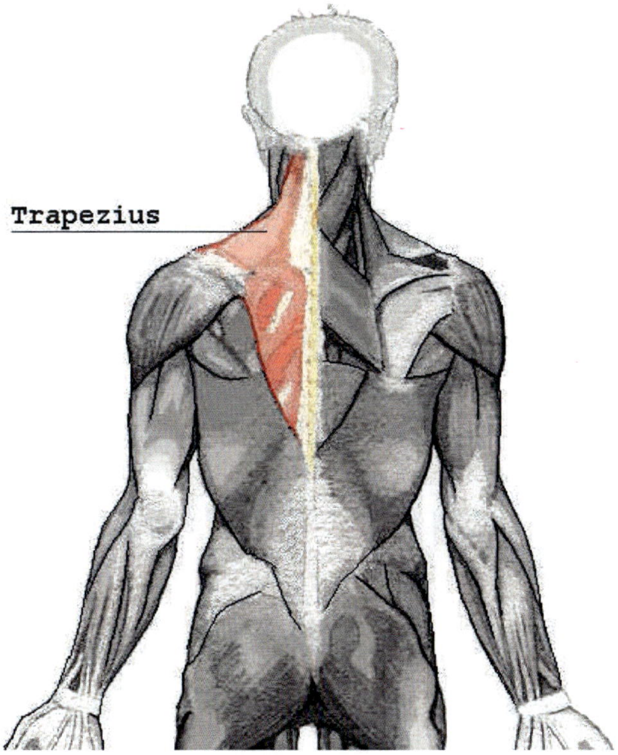

Figure 3.6.24 - Trapezius muscle

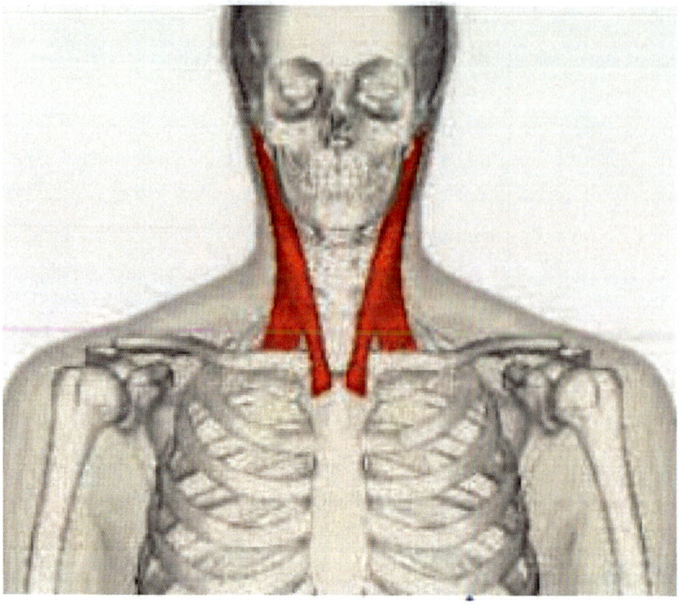

Figure 3.6.25 - Sternocleidomastoid muscle

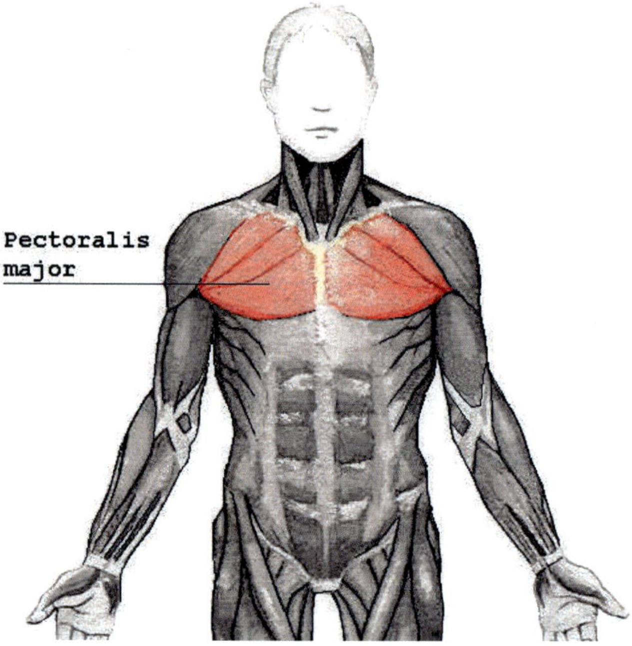

Figure 3.6.26 - Pectoralis major muscle

REVIEW QUESTIONS

1. An anesthesiologist is attempting to anesthetize the brachial plexus in the thoracic outlet. With relation to the posterior scalene and the sternocleidomastoid muscles, where should the injection be placed to approximate the brachial plexus?

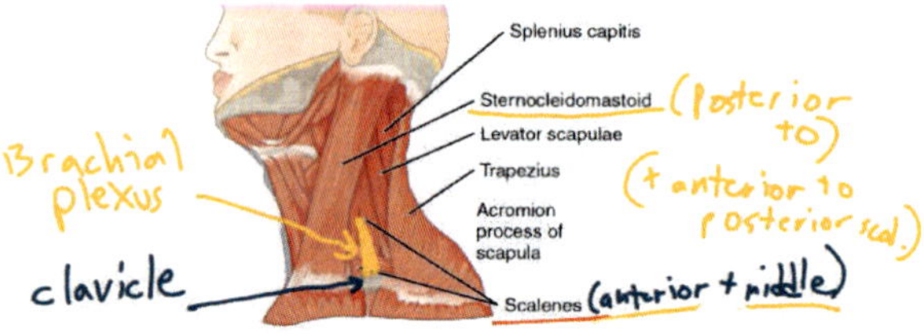

- **The brachial plexus runs between the anterior and middle scalene muscles. This means the brachial plexus would run posterior to the sternocleidomastoid muscle and anterior to the posterior scalene muscle.**

2. A 19-year-old female presents to the physician with upper arm pain following a sports injury. An MRI confirms the tear and a radiologist indicates the location with an arrow. The patient will most likely have difficulty with what movement?

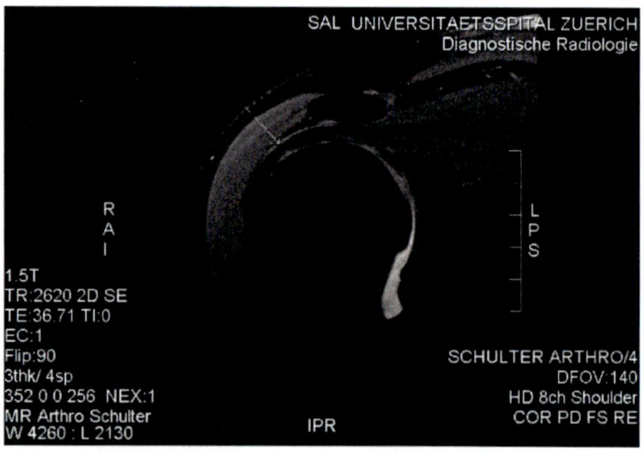

- **Answer: To reach the lateral side of the humeral head, the supraspinatus travels between the acromion and the head of the humerus. Supraspinatus dysfunction, or tear, would decrease its ability to abduct the shoulder from 0 to 15 degrees.**

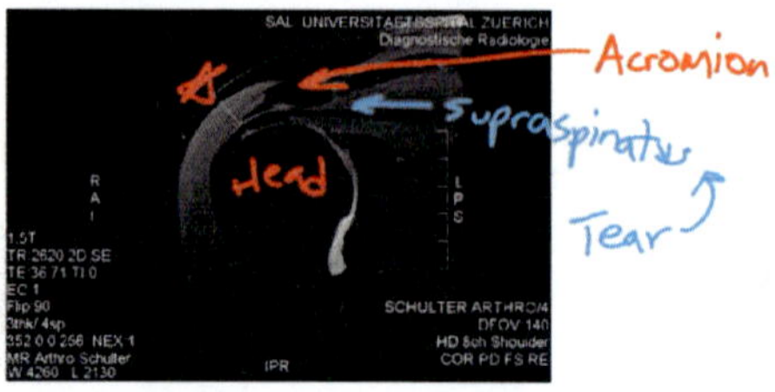

REVIEW QUESTIONS

3. A 15-year-old boy says his left arm feels weaker than normal after a biking accident. On exam, the boy is instructed to keep his upper limbs in the position shown below. The physician places her own hand against the boy's right palm and instructs the boy to push against her hand. He does this without difficulty. However, when the same action is performed with the boy's left arm, the boy cannot resist the physician's hand. This patient is most likely experiencing weakness in what muscle?

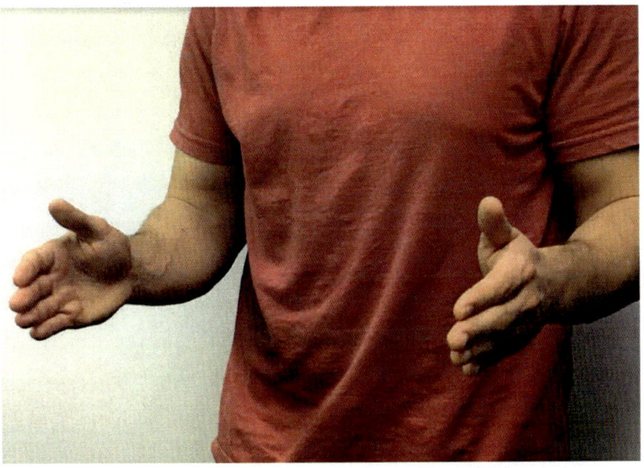

- **Answer: The patient is unable to perform internal rotation with his arm, which is performed by the subscapularis muscle.**
  - **Note: Remember the memory hook, Sub-I**

4. A 24-year-old male regularly performs the exercise shown below. The right image demonstrates muscular contraction. By performing this exercise, the patient is hoping to strengthen a muscle that attaches to the iliac crest as well as the humerus and spinous processes. What nerve innervates this muscle?

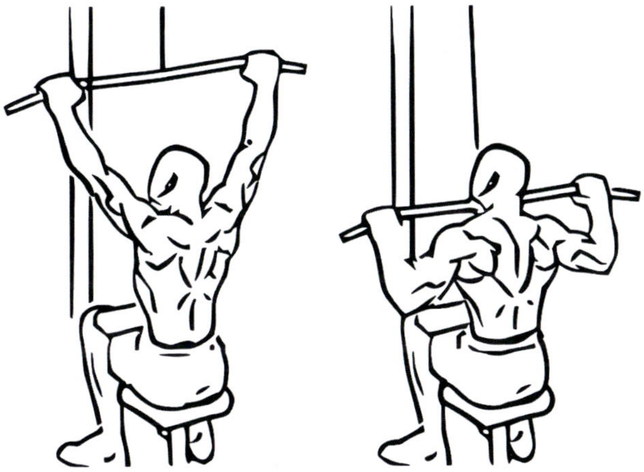

By Everkinetic (http://db.everkinetic.com/) [CC BY-SA 3.0 (https://creativecommons.org/licenses/by-sa/3.0)], via Wikimedia Commons

- **Answer: The latissimus dorsi performs this motion. The question stem states the muscle in question attaches to the iliac crest, several spinous processes on the vertebrae and the humerus, indicating the latissimus dorsi muscle. This muscle is innervated by the thoracodorsal nerve.**

Section V - Elbow and Wrist

I. There are four major landmarks to be familiar with regarding the elbow. See Table 3.6.6 showing the Elbow Landmarks.

Location	Pathology
Medial epicondyle	• Medial epicondylitis: repetitive flexion (forearm flexors attach to medial epicondyle) • Ulnar nerve damage
Lateral epicondyle	• Lateral epicondylitis: repetitive extension (forearm extensors attach to lateral epicondyle)
Supracondylar area	• Supracondylar fracture: median nerve damage
Annular ligament	• Radial head subluxation: stretching of extended and pronated arm → annular ligament slips superiorly → anterior subluxation of radial head

Table 3.6.6 - Elbow landmarks

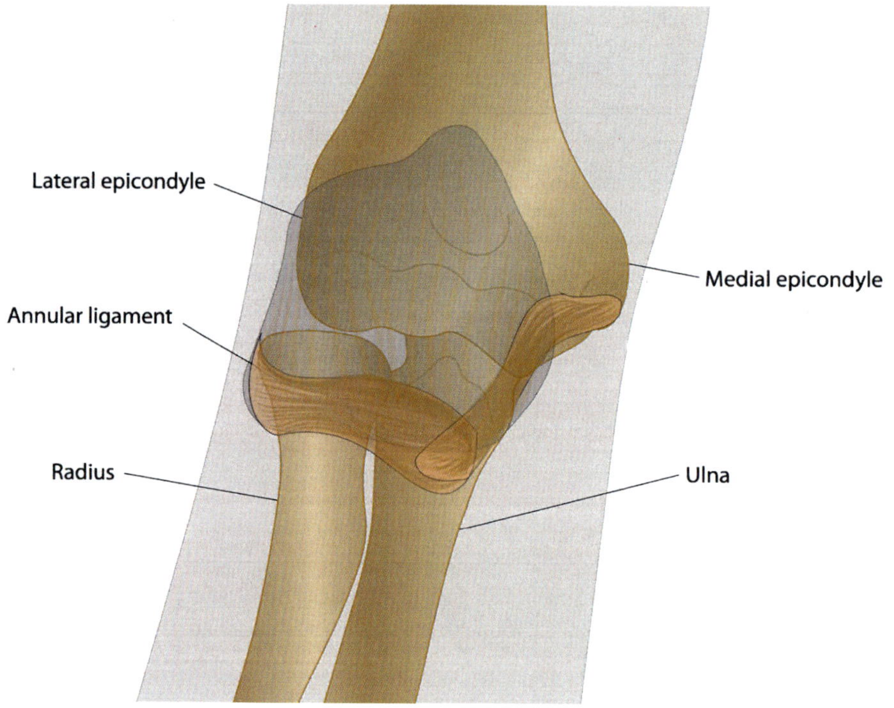

Figure 3.6.27 - Anterior elbow joint

II. Ulnar Nerve Palsy

A. The ulnar nerve runs posterior to the medial epicondyle.

B. Medial epicondyle damage can cause ulnar nerve dysfunction (palsy).

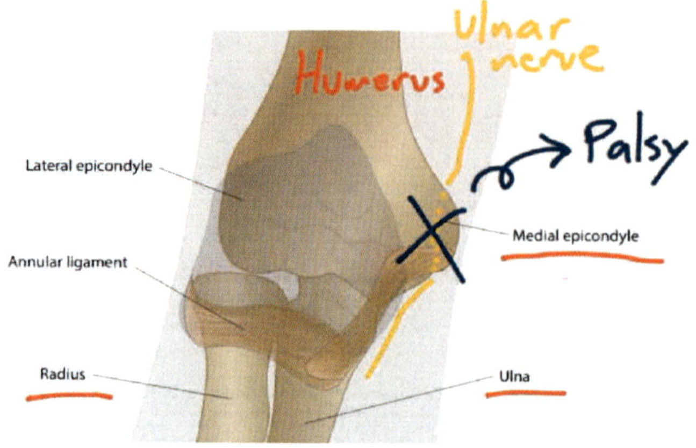

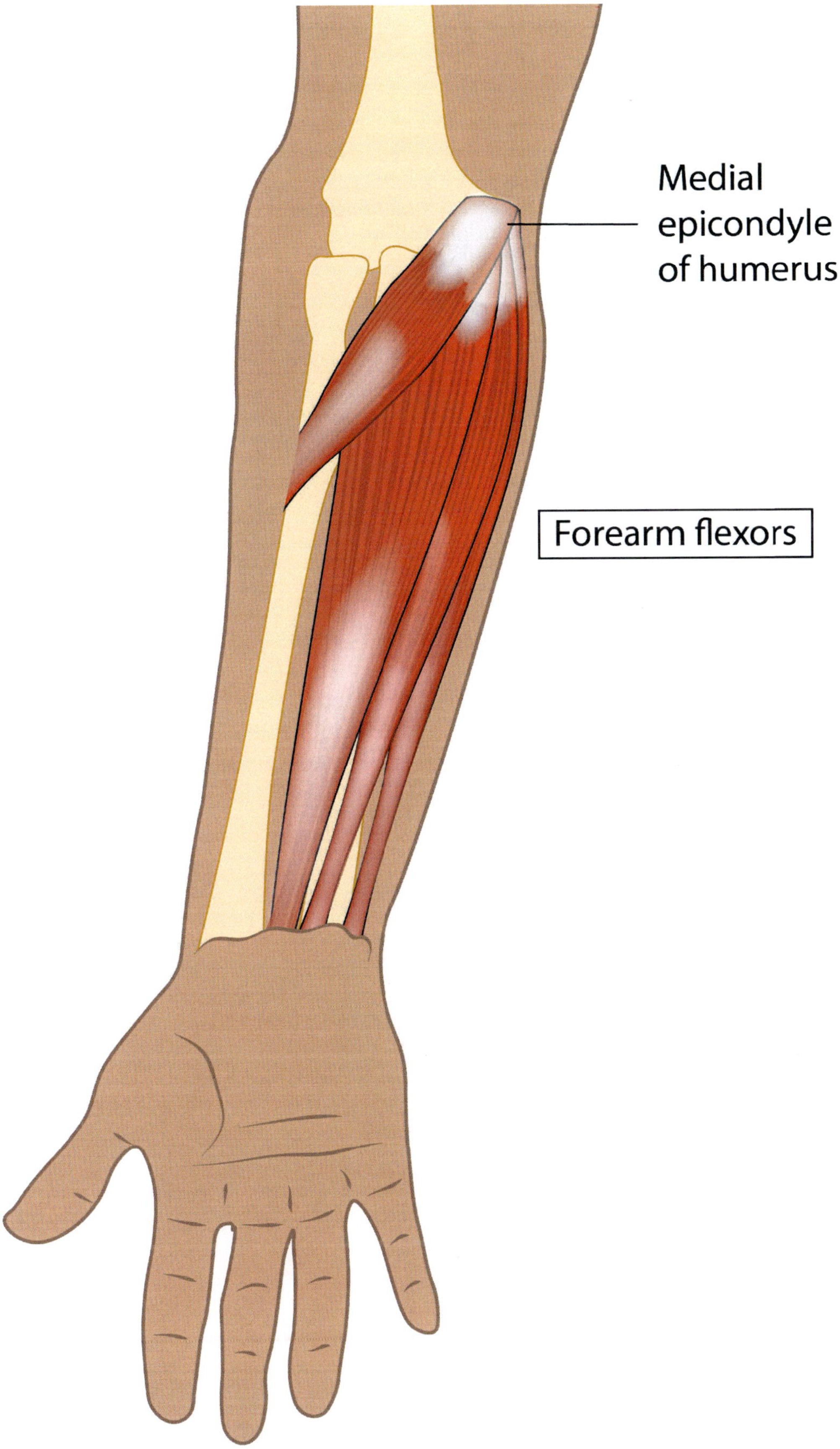

Figure 3.6.28 - Forearm flexors

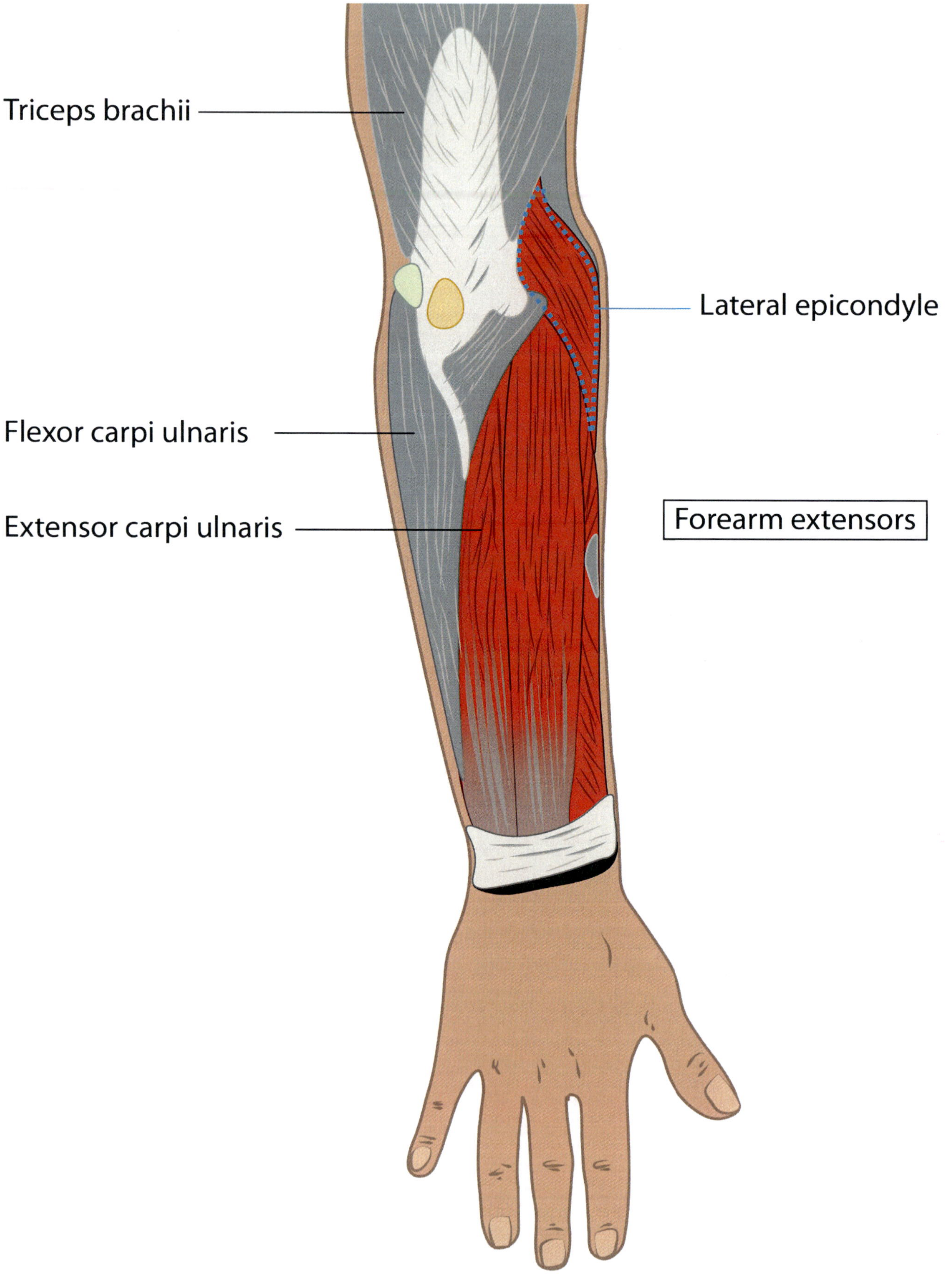

Figure 3.6.29 - Forearm extensors

III. Lateral Epicondylitis

A. Inflammation caused by overuse of forearm extensors.

B. The back hand motion is a common culprit.

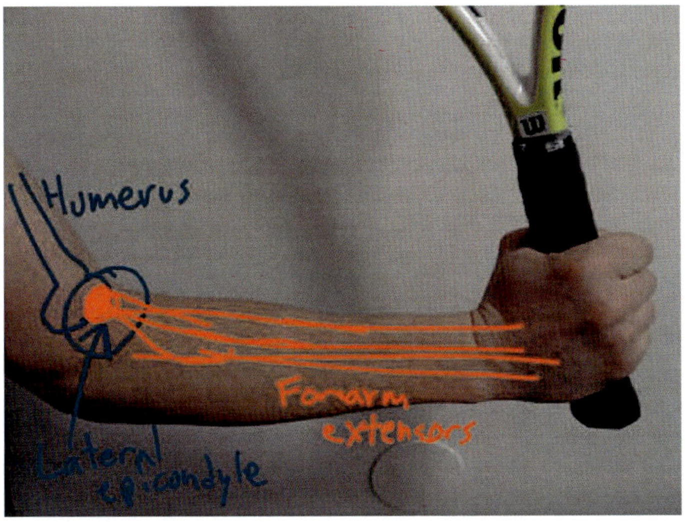

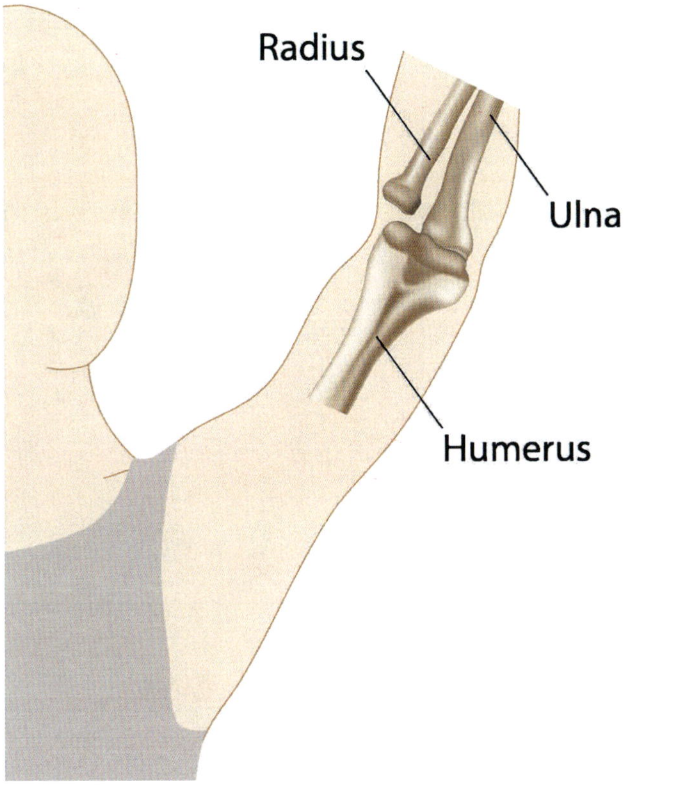

Figure 3.6.30 - Radial head subluxation

Location	Pathology
Scaphoid bone	• Fall fracture: dorsal scaphoid branch cannot supply proximal bone → avascular necrosis
Lunate bone	• Fall fracture: lunate dislocation → median nerve compression
Hamate (and Guyon's canal)	• Injury to hook of hamate → ulnar nerve palsy • Guyon's canal compression (handlebar compression) → ulnar nerve palsy
Carpal tunnel	• Carpal tunnel syndrome: repetitive use injury → median nerve palsy

Table 3.6.7 - Wrist landmarks

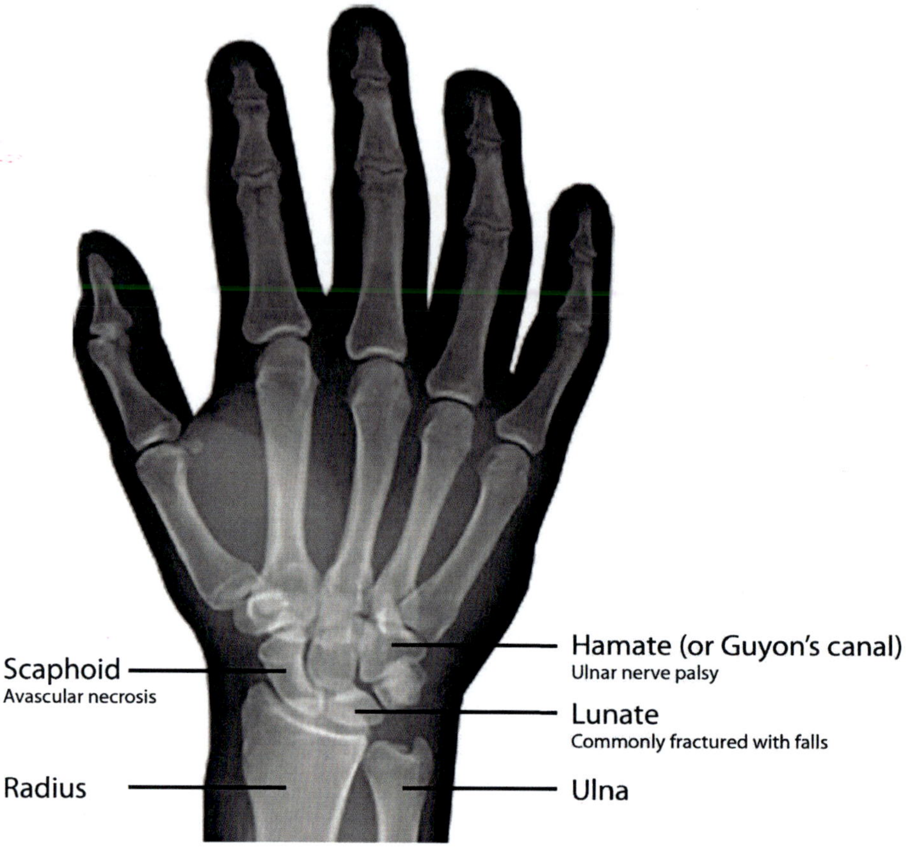

Figure 3.6.31 - Carpal bones

By Hellerhoff [CC BY-SA 3.0 (https://creativecommons.org/licenses/by-sa/3.0)], from Wikimedia Commons, adjustments made

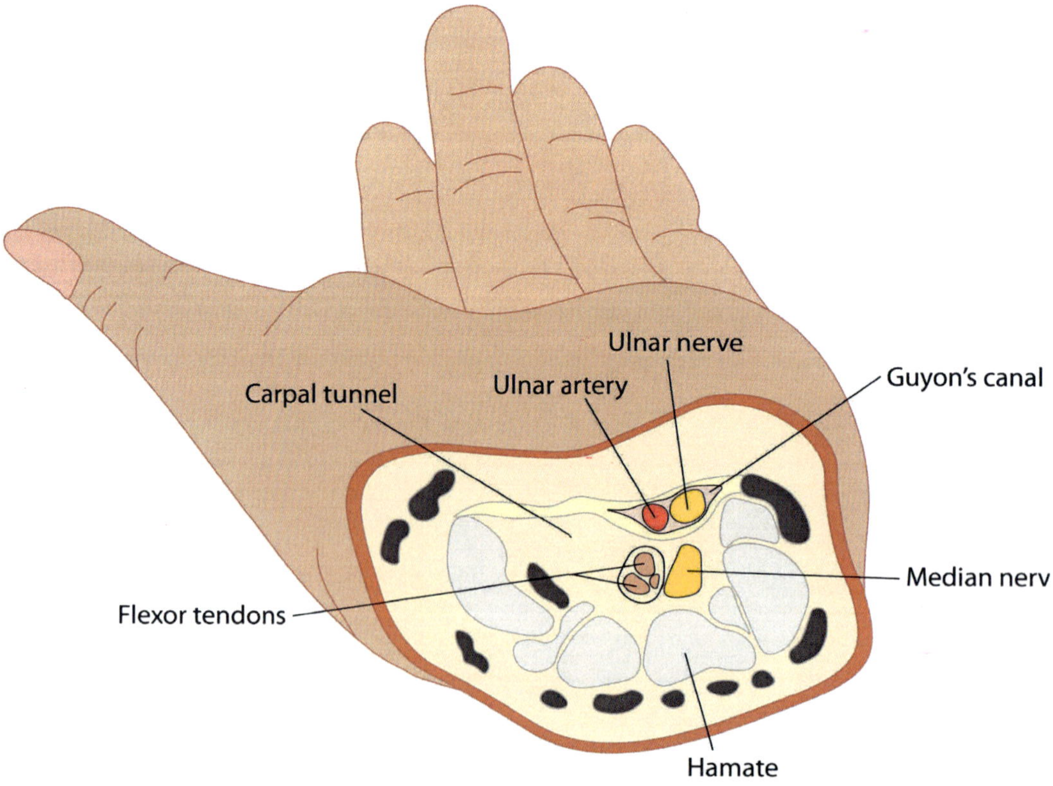

Figure 3.6.32 - Axial view of the wrist

REVIEW QUESTIONS

1. A 29-year-old military officer presents to the clinic for routine blood work. The phlebotomist palpates the arm in preparation for the procedure. The patient winces in pain when the area, labeled with a blue circle, is palpated. A nearby doctor suspects the pain is likely from an overuse injury. What innervates the forearm flexors?

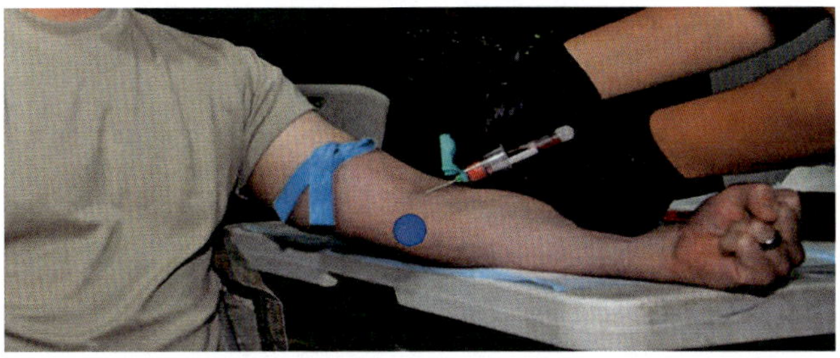

- **Answer: Hopefully you noticed that this is the medial epicondyle and the patient likely has medial epicondylitis**
- **Medial epicondylitis can occur with overuse of the forearm flexors that originate here**
- **Most of the forearm flexors are innervated by the median nerves; however, from our previous lecture on the median and ulnar nerve, we discussed that the flexor digitorum profundus is innervated by both the median and ulnar nerves, so you could say median nerve or the median and ulnar nerve, technically.**

2. A 9-year-old boy falls out of a tree and embraces the impact directly with the palm of his hand. What bones are commonly injured with this type of fall? What nerve may be injured?

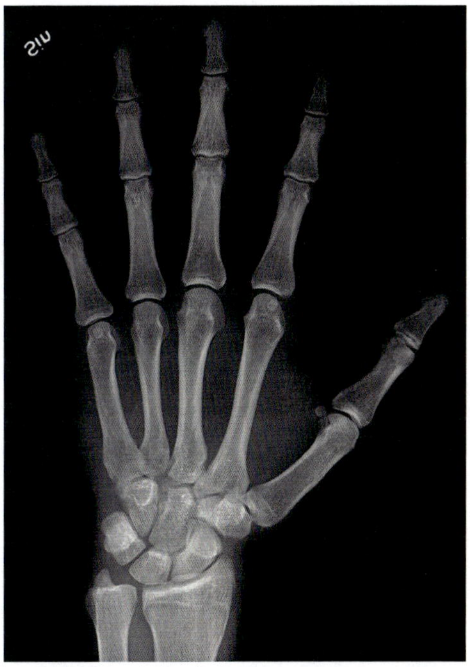

By Mikael Häggström [CC0], from Wikimedia Commons

- **Answer: A fall on an outstretched hand can fracture the radius and the two carpal bones that it articulates with: the lunate and the scaphoid bone. Damage to the scaphoid bone can result in avascular necrosis. Damage to the lunate bone can result in median nerve compression**

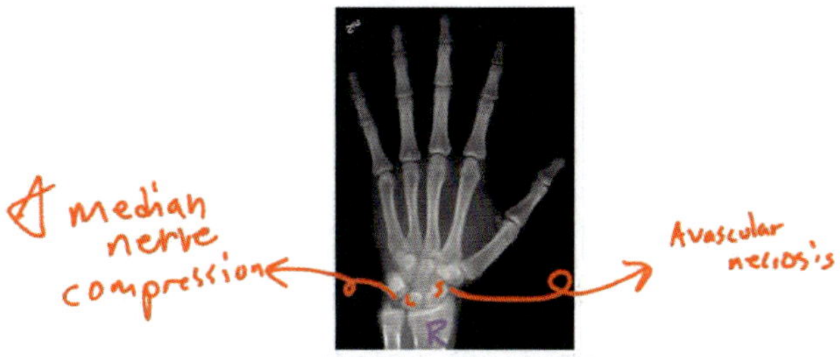

By Mikael Häggström [CC0], from Wikimedia Commons

Section VI - Lumbosacral Plexus

I. The lumbosacral plexus is a group of nerves emanating from the lumbar region that provides motor and sensory information to the trunk and lower extremities.

Nerve	Motor	Sensory	Cause of Injury/ Comments
Iliohypogastric (T12-L1)	• Thoracic and pelvic stability (transversus abdominis) • Rotation and torsion of the trunk (internal oblique)	• Suprapubic region	• Abdominal surgery (sutures of transverse incisions may trap nerve)
Genitofemoral (L1-L2)	• Cremaster reflux (cremaster)	• Scrotum (male) • Labia majora (female) • Medial thigh	• Abdominal surgery (retractor blades)
Lateral femoral cutaneous (L2-L3)	• N/A	• Anterolateral thigh	• Tight pants, surgery, obesity, or pregnancy • Compression results in meralgia paresthetica
Obturator (L2-L4)	• Hip adduction (adductor magnus, adductor brevis, adductor longus, gracilis, pectineus, and obturator externus)	• Medial thigh	• Pelvic trauma or bladder cancer
Femoral (L2-L4)	• Knee extension (quadriceps muscle group) • Hip flexion (quadriceps muscle group, iliacus, pectineus, and sartorius)	• Anterior thigh (anterior cutaneous branches) • Medial leg (saphenous nerve)	• Pelvic trauma or psoas muscle pathology • Anesthetize via injection at inguinal crease
Sciatic (L4-S3)	• Knee flexion (biceps femoris, semitendinosus, semimembranosus, and adductor magnus)	• See common peroneal and tibial sensory	• Vertebral disc herniation or posterior hip dislocation
Common Peroneal (L4-S2)	• Superficial: foot eversion (peroneus longus and peroneus brevis) • Deep: foot dorsiflexion (tibialis anterior)	• Superficial: dorsum of foot (except 1st web space) and lateral shin • Deep: 1st web space	• Fibular neck fracture or local compression (lateral decubitus position under anesthesia) • Memory hook: "foot dropPED"
Tibial (L4-S3)	• Toe flexion (flexor hallucis longus and flexor digitorum longus) • Foot inversion (tibialis posterior) • Foot plantarflexion (gastrocnemius, plantaris, and soleus)	• Sole of foot	• Knee trauma, popliteal (Baker) cyst, tarsal tunnel syndrome • Memory hook: "can't stand on TIPtoes"
Superior gluteal (L4-S1)	• Hip abduction and stabilization of the pelvis (gluteus medius, gluteus minimus, and tensor fascia latae)	• N/A	• Intramuscular injection to superomedial gluteal region • Trendelenburg sign • Gluteus medius lurch
Inferior gluteal (L5-S2)	• Hip extension (gluteus maximus)	• N/A	• Posterior hip dislocation
Pudendal (S2-S4)	• Pelvic floor sphincters (urethral and anal)	• Perineum	• Stretching during childbirth • Targeted for perineal anesthesia

Table 3.6.8 - Lumbosacral plexus

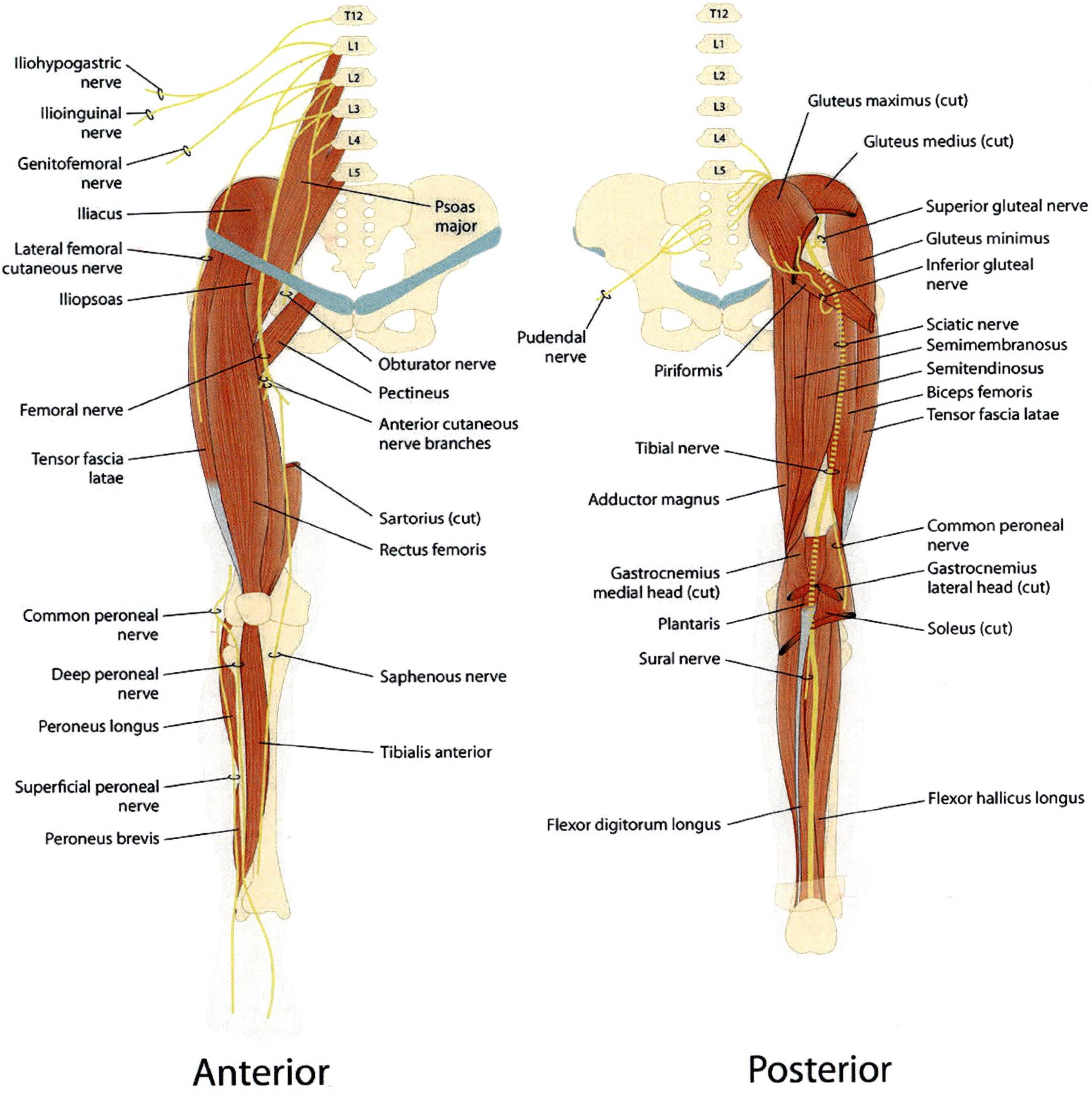

Figure 3.6.33 - Lumbosacral plexus

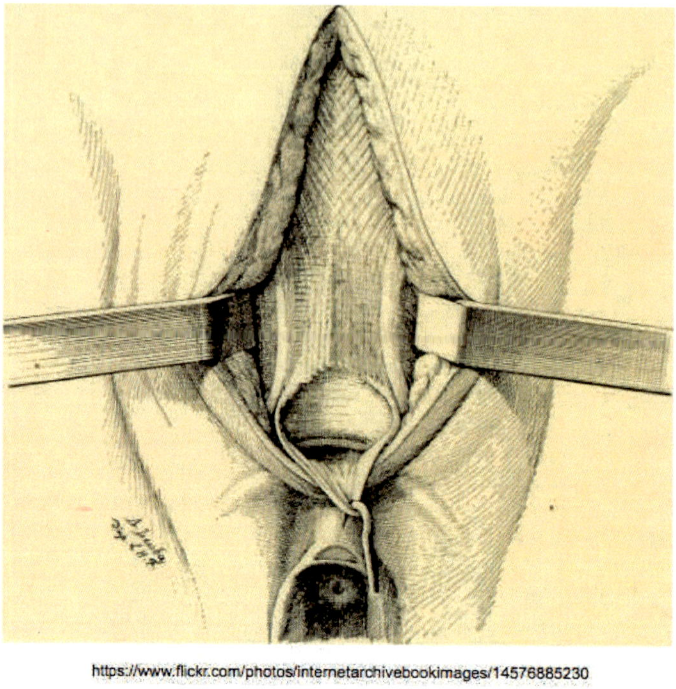

Figure 3.6.34 - Retractor blades

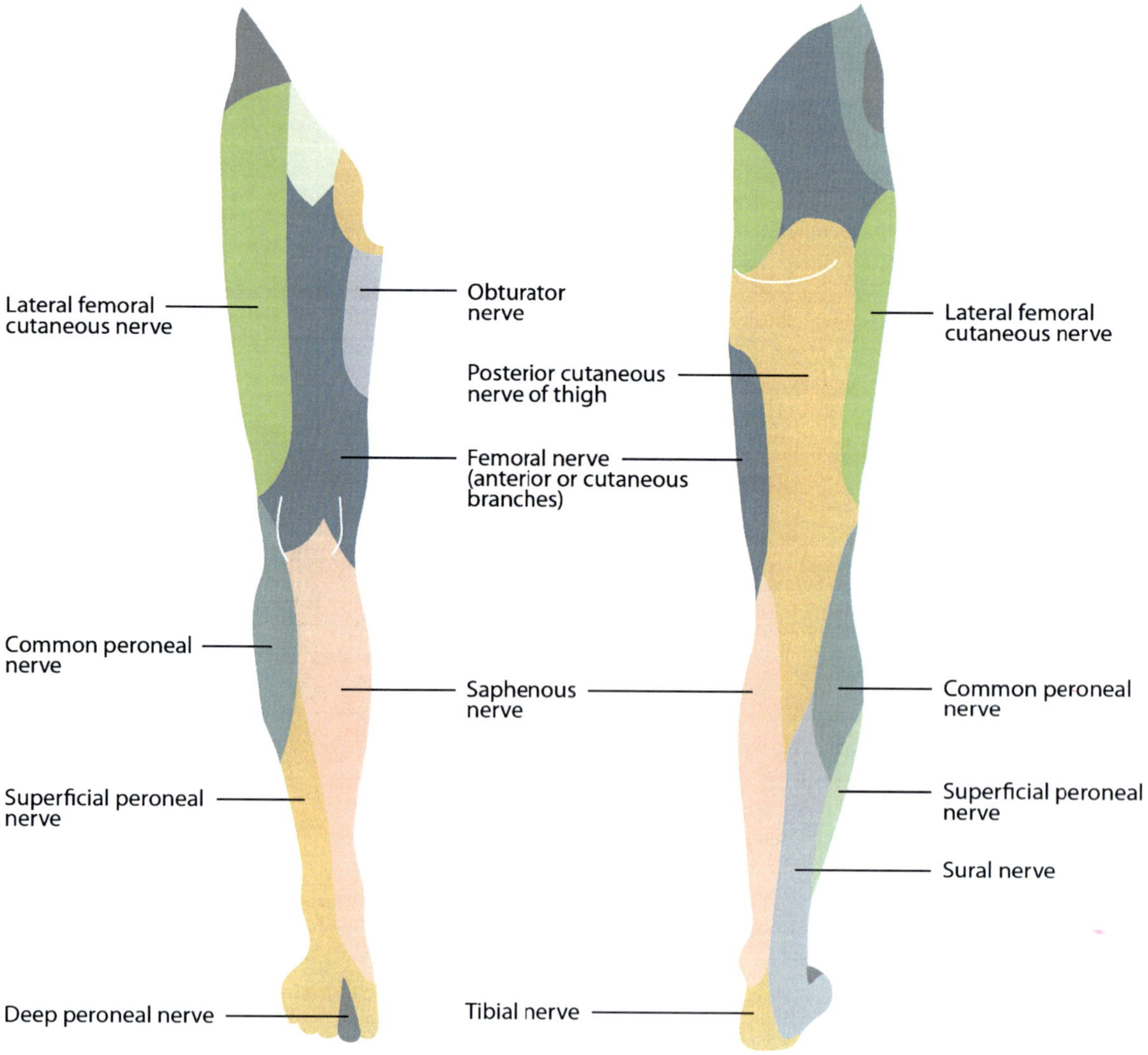

Figure 3.6.35 - Cutaneous innervation of the lower extremities

REVIEW QUESTIONS

1. A 42-year-old female presents to the emergency department due to flank pain and difficulty walking for the past several days. Walking upstairs has become particularly difficult for her. Her temperature is 38.6° C (101.5° F). Physical examination reveals right-sided weakness with knee extension and hip flexion. A CT scan shows an abscess near the right paraspinal muscles. What other finding on physical examination is most likely to be discovered in this individual?

   A) A diminished right patellar reflex
   B) Loss of sensation on the medial thigh of the right leg
   C) Impaired knee flexion of the right leg
   D) Loss of sensation on the lateral thigh of the right leg

- **Correct answer is A**
- **Right sided flank pain, a fever of 38.6° C, and a CT scan showing an abscess near paraspinal muscles → psoas muscle abscess**
- **Difficulty with knee extension and hip flexion → femoral nerve injury → diminished right patellar reflex (associated with L3-L4 region and the femoral nerve originates from the L2-L4 region)**
- **B is incorrect - the obturator nerve supplies sensory information to the medial thigh**
- **C is incorrect - the sciatic nerve is responsible for knee flexion**
- **D is incorrect - the lateral femoral cutaneous nerve supplies sensory information to the lateral thigh**

Spinal Cord Level	Reflex
C5-C6	Biceps reflex
C7-C8	Triceps reflex
L1-L2	Cremaster reflex
L3-L4	Patellar reflex
S1-S2	Achilles reflex
S3-S4	Anal wink reflex

2. A 19-year-old male is brought to the emergency department after injuring his left knee in a motor vehicle accident. Physical examination reveals a moderate level of pain over the leg but no motor or sensory deficits. An x-ray of the left leg shows several small fractures in the distal femur and proximal tibia. After thorough evaluation he is placed in a cast that spans the length of his entire leg. At a follow-up appointment 4 days later he is unable to evert and dorsiflex the left foot but the pain has diminished. Which of the following most likely explains these findings?

   A) A nerve was injured in the motor vehicle accident
   B) Limb compartment syndrome
   C) Medial tibial stress syndrome
   D) A nerve was compressed

- **Correct answer is D**
- **The patient didn't experience motor or sensory deficits immediately after the accident**
- **He was placed in a cast for 4 days and THEN experienced weakness**
- **Inability to evert and dorsiflex the left foot → left common peroneal nerve injury due to nerve compression**
- **A is incorrect - physical examination after the accident didn't show any motor or sensory deficits. The deficits only occurred several days later after the cast was applied.**
- **B is incorrect - This is associated with severe pain and a swollen leg which this patient did not have at his follow up visit.**
- **C is incorrect - this is also known as shin splints which presents with pain and tenderness over the anterior aspect of the leg. It's commonly associated with runners.**

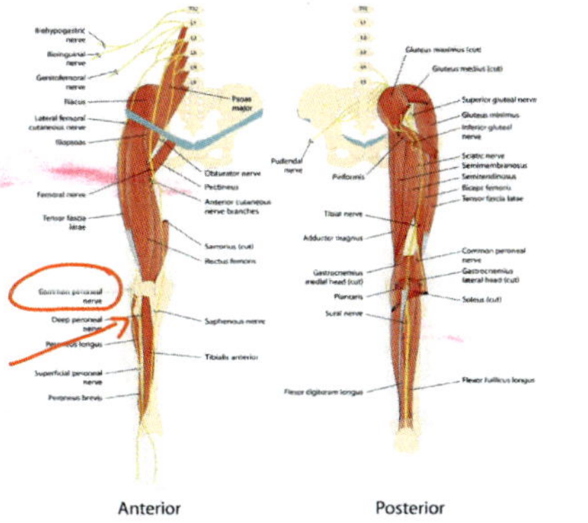

Section VII - Hip

I. The hip joint
   A. The hip joint is formed between the acetabulum and the femur
   B. Hip flexors: iliacus, iliopsoas, sartorius, and tensor fasciae latae muscles
      1. The psoas major muscle facilitates back flexion
   C. Hip extensors: gluteus maximus, semitendinosus, semimembranosus, and biceps femoris muscles
   D. Hip adductors: adductor magnus, adductor brevis, adductor longus, gracilis, and pectineus muscles
   E. Hip abductors: gluteus medius and gluteus minimus muscles

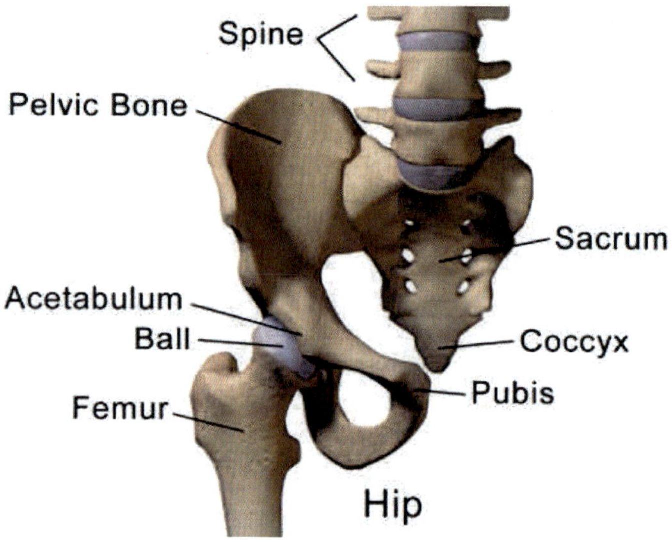

Figure 3.6.36 - Hip bones
BruceBlaus [CC BY 3.0 (https://creativecommons.org/licenses/by/3.0)], from Wikimedia Commons

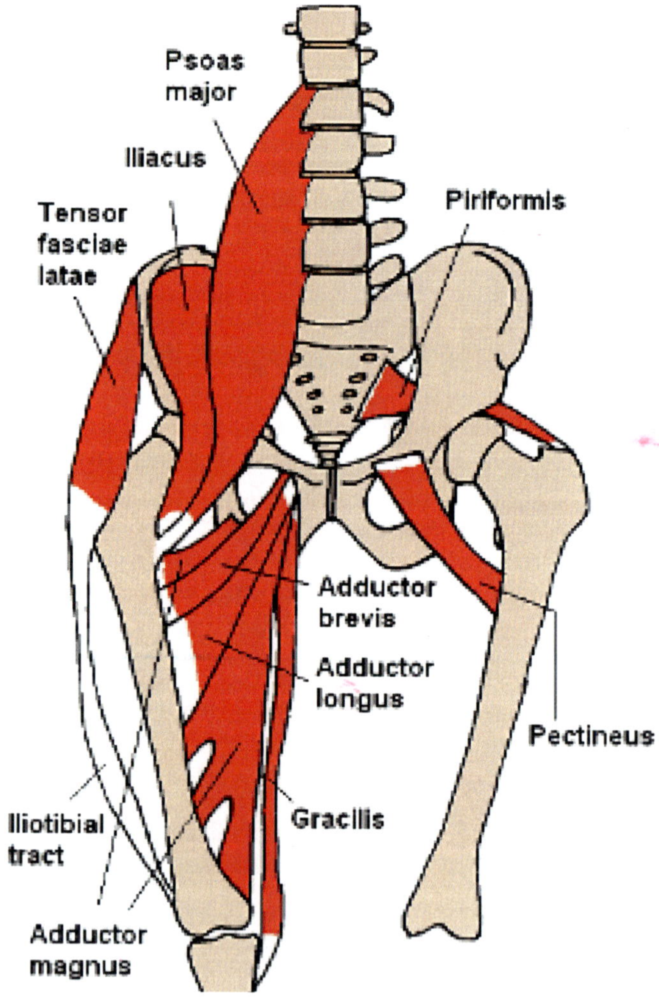

Figure 3.6.36 - Hip muscles
Beth Ohara (CC BY-SA 370 (http://creativecommons.org/licenses/by-sa/3.0/)), from Wikimedia Commons

II. Nerve injuries

A. The superior gluteal nerve

1. Originates from the L4-S1 region
2. Provides motor information responsible for hip abduction and stabilization of the pelvis
3. Innervates the gluteus medius, gluteus minimus, and tensor fasciae latae muscles
4. Injured due to an improperly placed intramuscular injection → positive Trendelenburg sign and gluteus medius lurch

B. The Trendelenburg sign

1. Hip contralateral to the injured nerve drops when standing on one foot

C. Gluteus medius lurch

1. The patient leans towards the ipsilateral injury while walking to compensate for pelvic instability

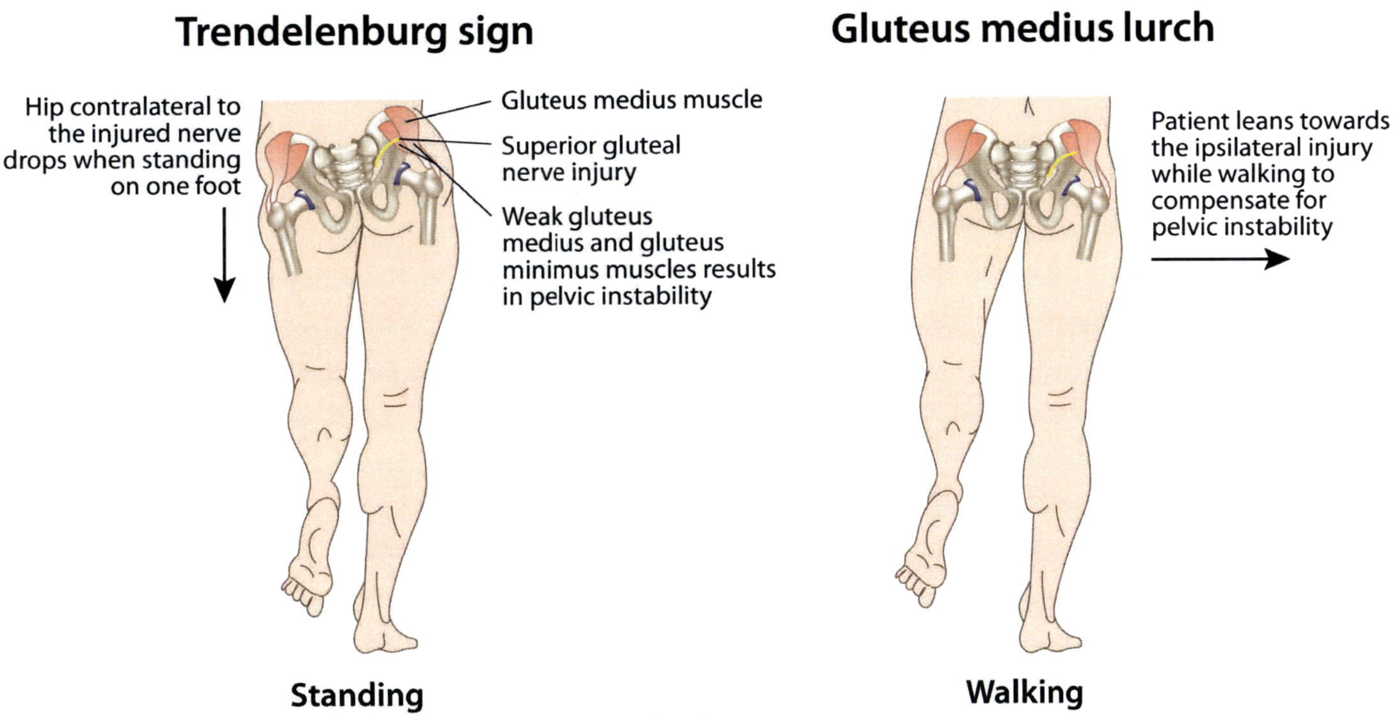

Figure 3.6.38 - Trendelenburg sign and gluteus medius lurch

D. The inferior gluteal nerve

1. Originates from the L5-S2 region
2. Provides motor information responsible for hip extension
3. Innervates the gluteus maximus muscle
4. Injured due to a posterior hip dislocation

III. Trochanteric bursitis

A. Inflammation and pain lateral to the greater trochanter of the femur

B. Gluteal tendon and bursa involvement

C. Treatment includes heat, stretches, and NSAIDs

IV. Developmental dysplasia of the hip

A. Acetabulum development in newborns is disrupted → hip instability

B. Ortolani and Barlow maneuvers can be helpful in making a diagnosis

C. Diagnosis confirmed with ultrasound (cartilage doesn't ossify until ~4-6 months so x-ray cannot be used)

D. Treatment includes splints/harnesses

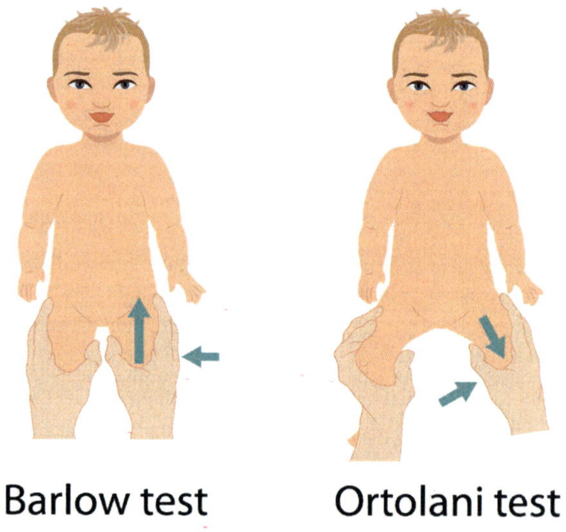

Figure 3.6.39 - Ortolani and Barlow maneuvers

V. Slipped capital femoral epiphysis (SCFE)

A. Often seen in obese adolescents

B. Fracture through growth plate → displaced epiphysis

C. Presents with hip/knee pain and an altered gait

D. Diagnosed using x-ray

E. Treatment includes surgery

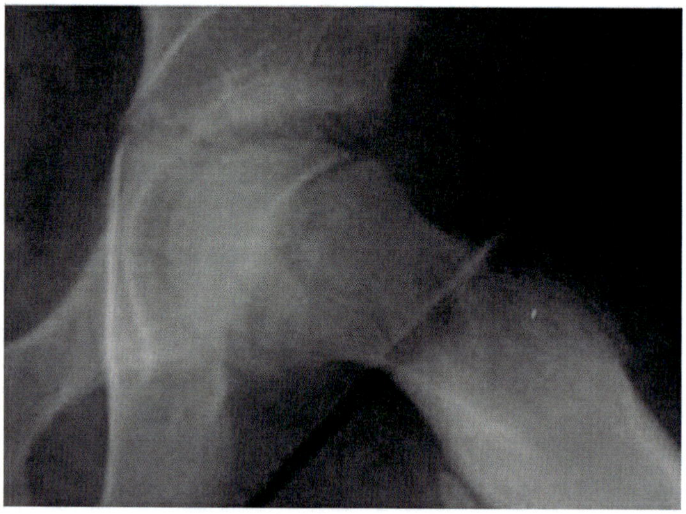

Mikir at English Wikipedia [Public domain], via Wikimedia Commons

Figure 3.6.40 - Slipped capital femoral epiphysis

VI. Legg-Calvé-Perthes disease

A. Avascular necrosis of the head of the femur

B. Often see in children between the ages of 5-7

C. Presents with hip pain and difficulty walking

D. 4:1 male to female ratio

E. Initial x-ray is frequently normal

REVIEW QUESTIONS

1. A 59-year-old female presents to the office due to hip pain. She has a history of osteoarthritis which has been refractory to nonsteroidal anti-inflammatory drugs. The physician performs a deep intramuscular injection in attempt to alleviate the pain. The patient returns to the clinic the next day due to difficulty walking. When asked to stand on the left leg, her right hip dips downward. Where was the injection most likely placed that resulted in this patient's condition?

    A) Inferomedial aspect of the left buttock
    B) Inferomedial aspect of the right buttock
    C) Superolateral aspect of the left buttock
    D) Superolateral aspect of the right buttock
    E) Superomedial aspect of the left buttock
    F) Superomedial aspect of the right buttock

- **Correct answer is E**
- **Improper placement of intramuscular injection in the buttock → injury to the superior gluteal nerve → positive Trendelenburg sign**
- **The superior gluteal nerve emerges above the piriformis muscle and terminates near the superomedial quadrant of the buttock**
- **If an injection is placed too far superomedially then the nerve may injured resulting in a positive Trendelenburg sign**
- **When asked to stand on the left leg, her right hip dips downward → left superior gluteal nerve injury**
- **A and B are incorrect - the inferomedial aspect of the buttock can damage the sciatic nerve due to its large size, but this would not result in a positive Trendelenburg sign**
- **C and D are incorrect - the superolateral aspect of the buttock is the ideal location for these types of injections so these would have not resulted in a positive Trendelenburg sign**
- **F is incorrect - the patient would have presented with a positive Trendelenburg sign on the opposite side**

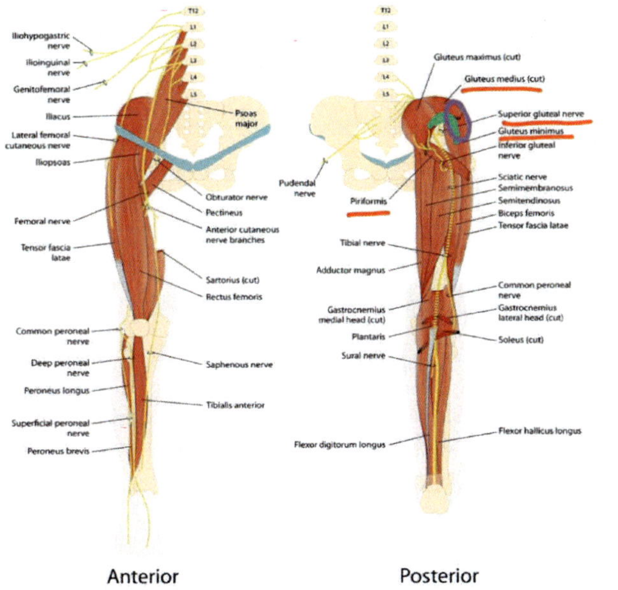

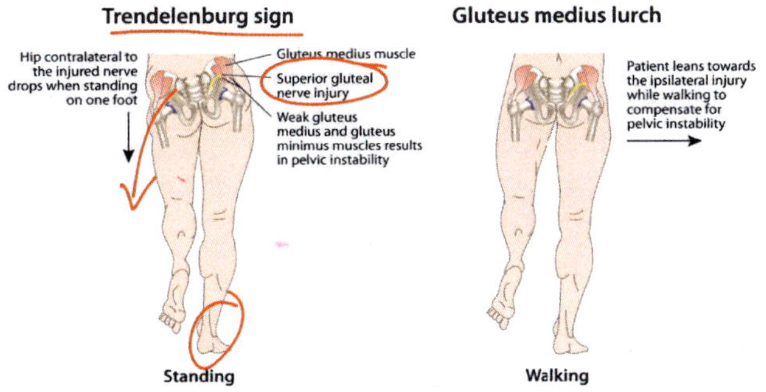

Section VIII - Lumbar Radiculopathy

I. Radiculopathy

A. A range of symptoms due to pinching of a nerve root as it exits the vertebral column

B. Most commonly due to a herniated disc

C. Spinal stenosis is a less common cause

D. Symptoms often include numbness, weakness, pain, and altered reflexes

II. Spinal Stenosis

A. Caused by narrowing of the central canal → nerve root compression → radiculopathy (especially when standing)

B. Hypertrophy of the ligamentum flavum

C. Age-related (disc degeneration)

D. Facet joint arthropathy

E. May also occur as a result of spondylolisthesis (slippage of a vertebra)

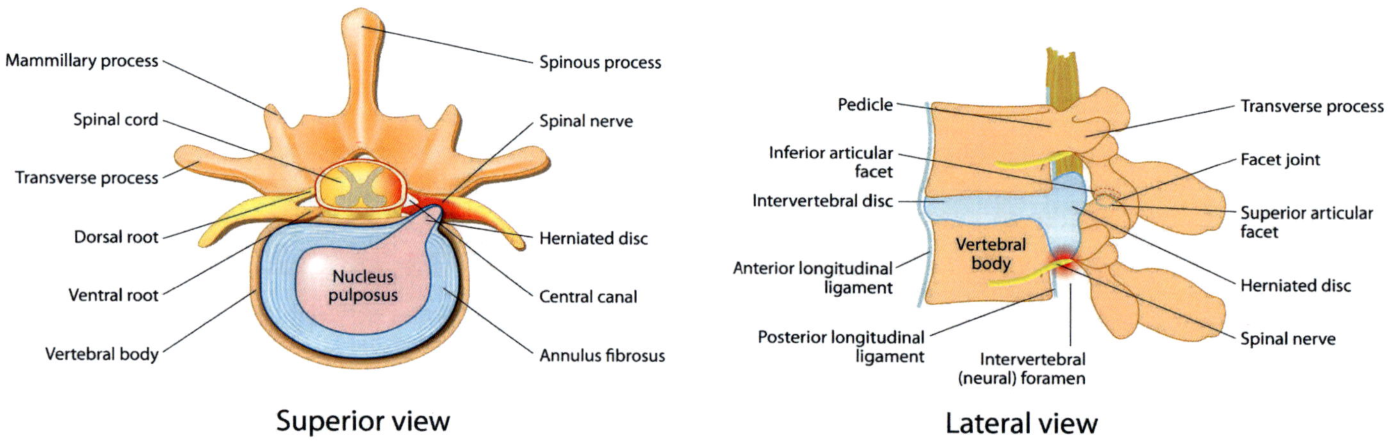

Figure 3.6.41 - Radiculopathy

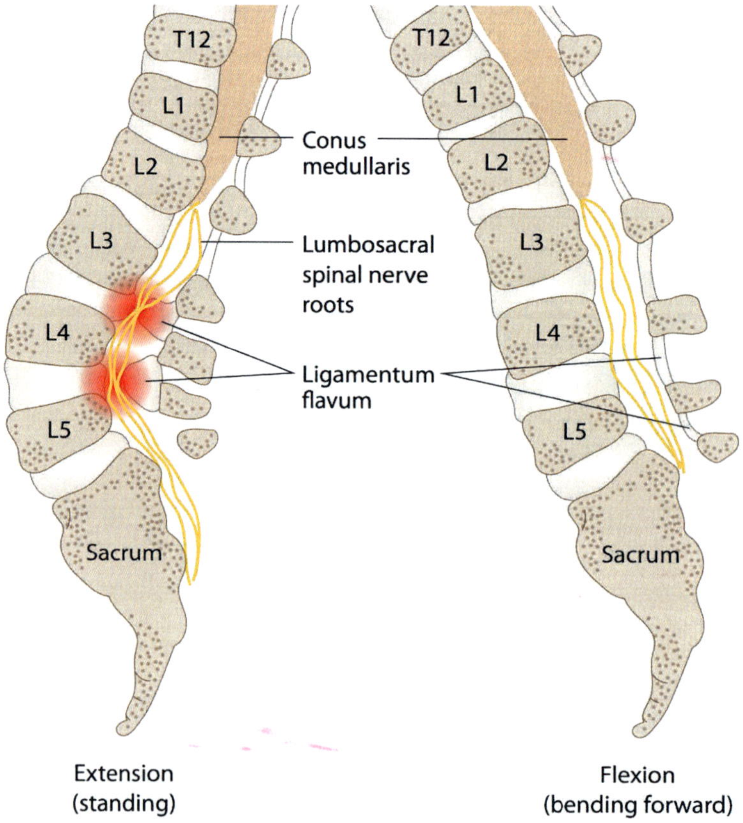

Figure 3.6.42 - Spinal stenosis

III. Sciatica

A. The sciatic nerve originates from the L4-S3 region

B. If the nerve roots are compressed at these regions it can result in symptoms of radiculopathy along the distribution of the sciatic nerve.

C. Dermatome and myotome levels as well as clinical reflexes provide clues about what nerve root is injured.

D. A positive straight leg test is indicative of lumbar radiculopathy

Spinal Cord Level	Reflex
C2	Posterior scalp
C3	Upper neck
C4	Lower neck
C6	1st digit (thumb)
C7	3rd digit (middle finger)
C8	5th digit (little finger)
T4	Nipple line
T7	Xiphoid process
T10	Navel line
L1	Inguinal ligament
L4	Patella and medial malleolus
L5	Dorsum of foot
S1	Lateral malleolus
S2-S4	Perineal region

Table 3.6.9 - Dermatomes

Spinal Cord Level	Reflex
C5	Shoulder abduction
C6	Elbow flexion
C7	Elbow extension
C8	Wrist flexion
T1	Thumb opposition
L2	Hip flexion
L3	Hip adduction
L4	Knee extension
L5	Ankle dorsiflexion
S1	Ankle plantar flexion
S2-S4	Erection

Table 3.6.10 - Myotomes

Spinal Cord Level	Reflex
C5-C6	Biceps reflex
C7-C8	Triceps reflex
L1-L2	Cremaster reflex
L3-L4	Patellar reflex
S1-S2	Achilles reflex
S3-S4	Anal wink reflex

Table 3.6.11 - Clinical reflexes

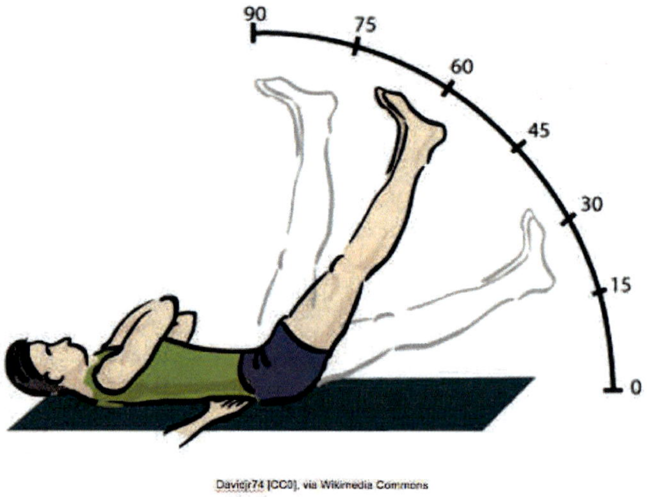

Figure 3.6.43 - Straight leg test

REVIEW QUESTIONS

?

1. A 27-year-old male presents to the office due to back pain which began suddenly yesterday morning while working in his garden. He states that the pain starts near his buttock region and radiates down the left lateral aspect of his leg. On physical exam, straight leg testing is positive on the left. Left foot dorsiflexion is weaker when compared to the right. There is also sensory loss along the dorsum of the foot. A herniated disc at what level is most likely responsible for this patient's condition?

   A) L4-L5
   B) L5-S1
   C) S1-S2
   D) S2-S3
   E) S3-S4

- **Correct answer is A**
- **Working in garden → herniated disc → sciatica (pain that radiates down the left lateral aspect of his leg)**
- **The L5 dermatome is associated with the dorsum of the foot**
- **The L5 myotome is associated with dorsi-flexion of the foot**
- **A herniated disc protrudes posterolaterally and inferiorly so an L4-L5 herniated disc → compression of the L5 nerve root**
- **B, C, D, and E would have resulted in different findings corresponding to their respective myotomes and dermatomes.**

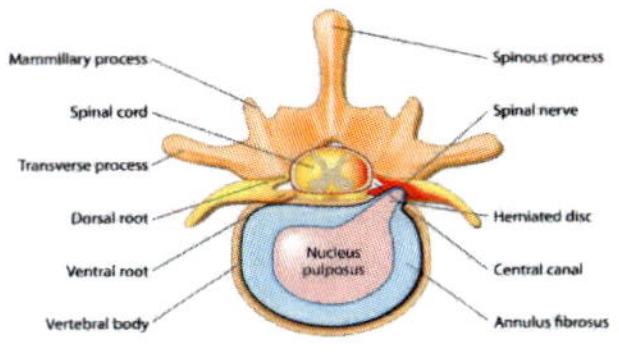

Superior view

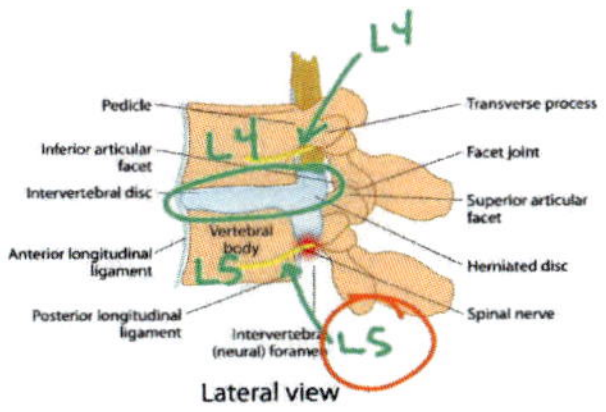

Lateral view

Section IX - Knee Ligaments and Menisci

I. For Step 1 you will most commonly be tested on the knee anatomy with regards to the ligaments, physical exam maneuvers, and corresponding imaging.

Structure	Anatomy	Injury	Physical Exam Maneuver
Anterior cruciate ligament (ACL)	• Lateral femoral condyle → anterior tibia (resists anterior force placed on the tibia)	• Injured following sudden decelerations or pivots while the knee extended (non-contact sports)	• Anterior drawer test • Lachman test
Posterior cruciate ligament (PCL)	• Medial femoral condyle → posterior tibia (resists posterior force placed on the tibia)	• Injured following a blow directed at the anterior proximal tibia (contact sports or motor vehicle accidents)	• Posterior drawer test
Medial collateral ligament (MCL)	• Medial epicondyle of the femur → medial condyle of the tibia (resists valgus stress)	• Injured following a blow to the lateral knee while the foot is planted or after a twisting motion	• Valgus stress test
Lateral collateral ligament (LCL)	• Lateral femoral condyle → head of the fibula (resists varus stress)	• Injured following a blow to the medial knee while the foot is planted	• Varus stress test
Menisci	• Fibrocartilage between the femur and tibia (reduces contact/friction between the femur and tibia)	• Twisting injury or due to chronic degenerative changes in elderly patients	• McMurray test

Table 3.6.12 - The knee

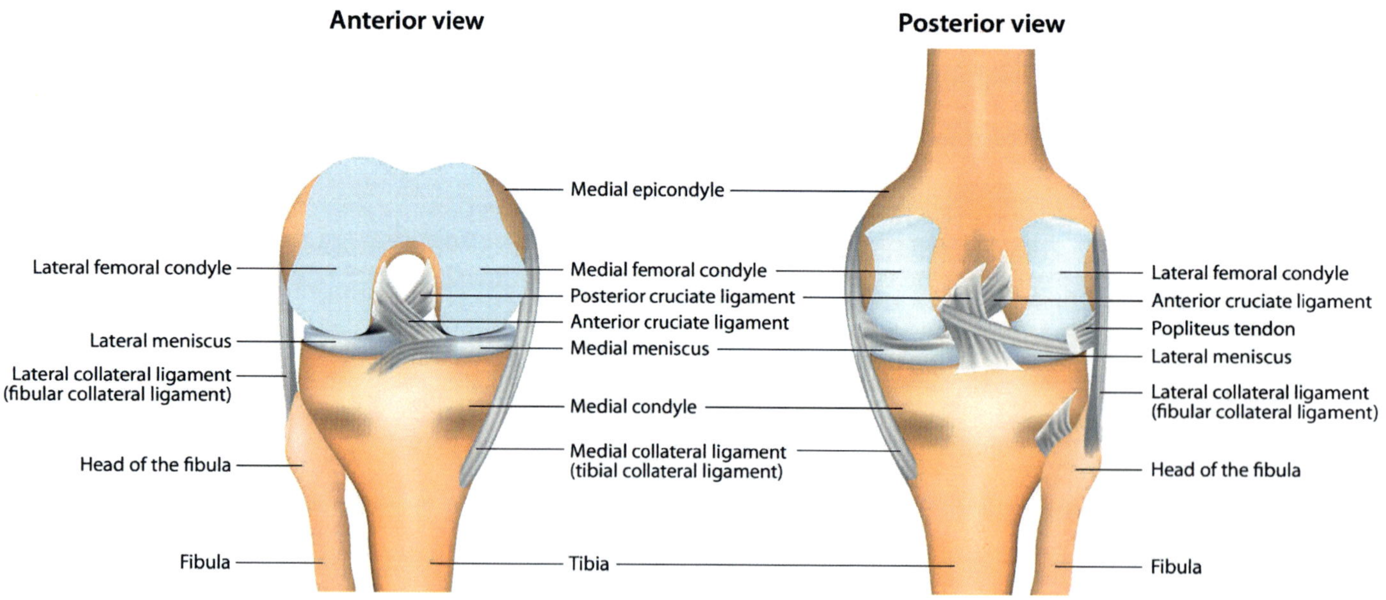

Figure 3.6.44 - Knee ligaments and menisci

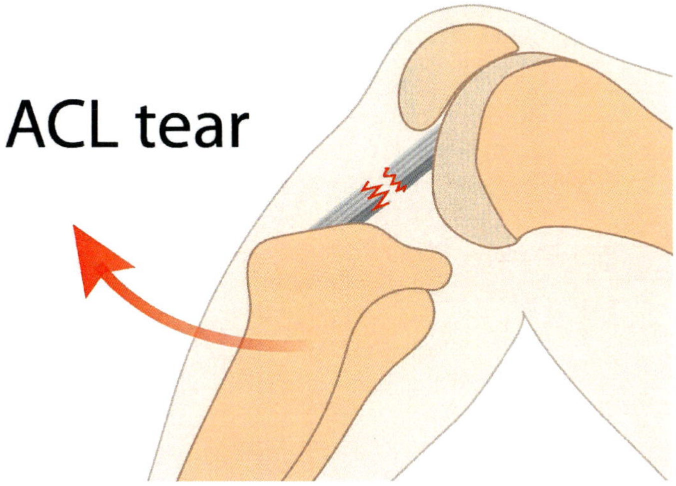

Figure 3.6.45 - Anterior drawer test

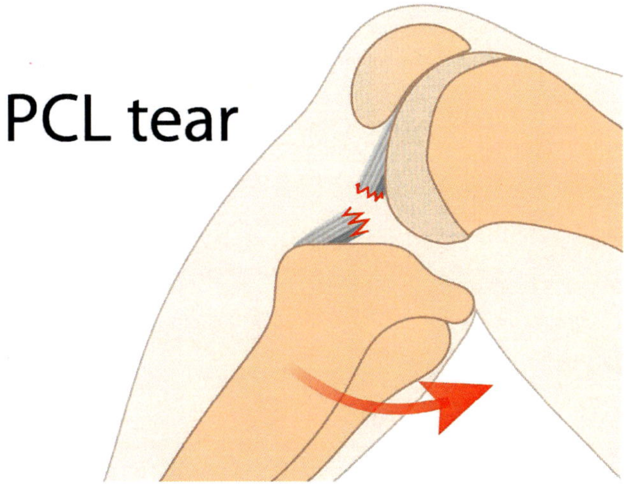

Figure 3.6.46 - Posterior drawer test

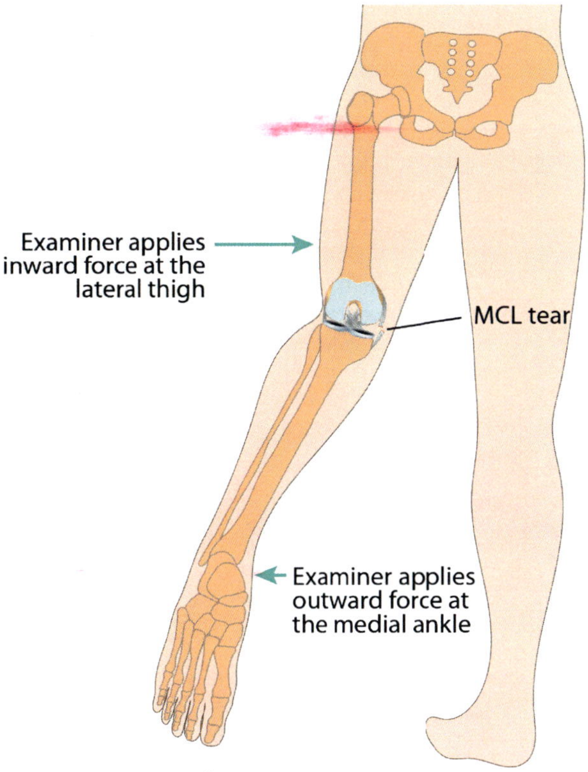

Figure 3.6.47 - Valgus stress test

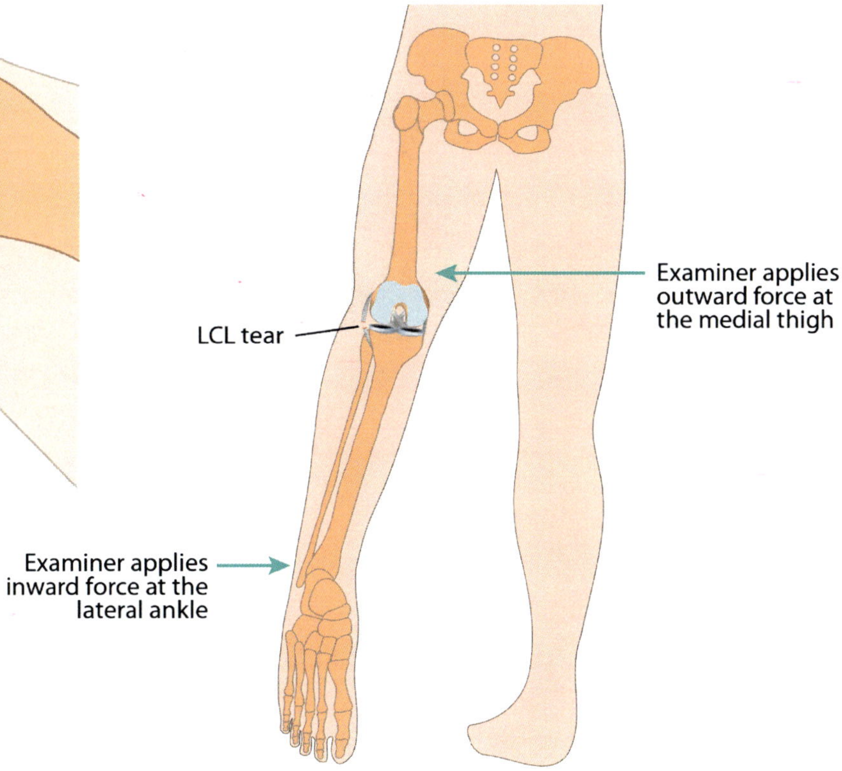

Figure 3.6.48 - Varus stress test

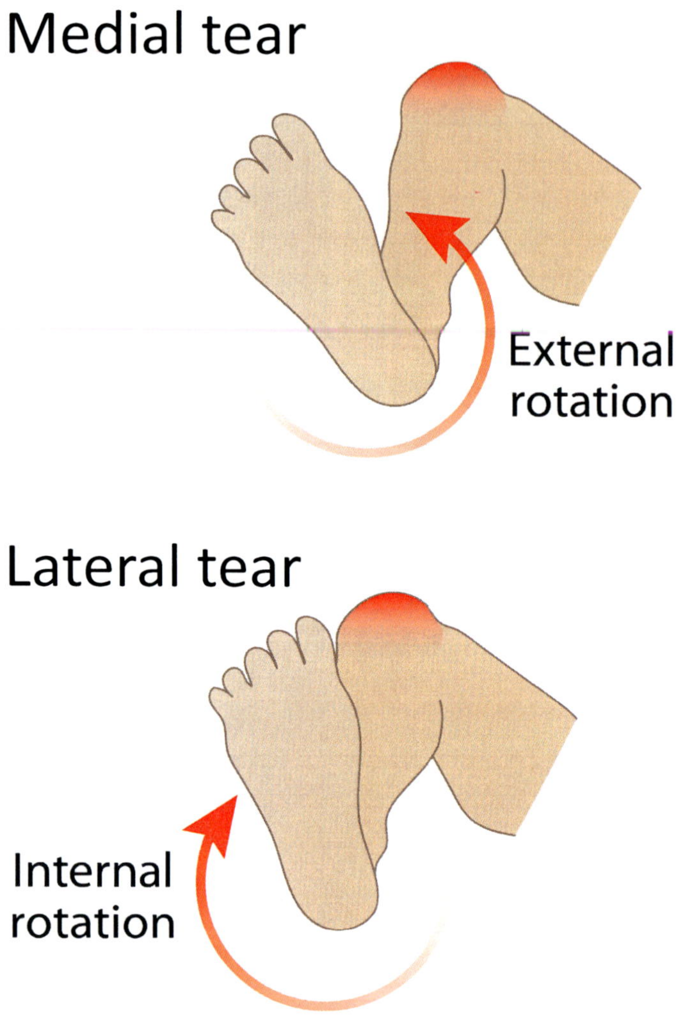

Figure 3.6.49 - McMurray test

REVIEW QUESTIONS

1. A 24-year-old male comes to the office due to knee pain following a flag football game. He states that as he attempted to catch the ball, the anterior aspect of his leg collided with another player. Physical examination reveals laxity of the tibia in relation to the femur when the knee is bent to 90 degrees and an anterior force is applied on the tibia in a backward motion. The ligament that is most likely injured attaches to which of the following structures?

    A) Medial condyle of the tibia
    B) Lateral femoral condyle
    C) Anterior tibia
    D) Medial femoral condyle

- **Correct answer is D**
- **The anterior aspect of the patient's leg collided with another player → contact sports injury → suggestive of a PCL injury**
- **Positive posterior drawer test → PCL injury**
- **A is incorrect - this is the attachment of the MCL**
- **B is incorrect - this is the attachment of the LCL**
- **C is incorrect - this is the attachment of the ACL**

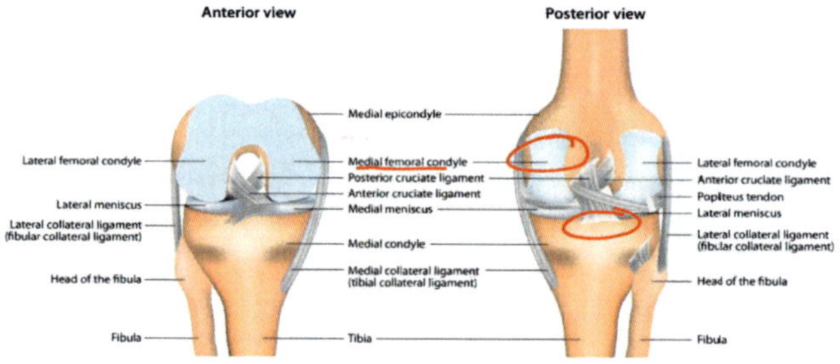

Section X - Other Knee and Leg Conditions

Condition	Definition	Etiology	Notes
Prepatellar bursitis	• Inflammation of the bursa anterior to the patella (prepatellar bursa)	• Trauma or pressure from repetitive kneeling	
Patellar fracture	• Partial or complete break in the patella bone	• Trauma to the knee	• Presents with a decreased ability to extend the knee (quadriceps tendon is unable to properly transmit force)
Iliotibial band syndrome	• Overuse injury involving the lateral knee where the iliotibial band crosses the lateral femoral epicondyle	• Friction between the iliotibial band and the lateral femoral epicondyle	• Common in runners
Osgood-Schlatter disease (traction apophysitis)	• Overuse injury involving the anterior knee which presents with progressive knee pain	• Repetitive strain and avulsion of the tibial tubercle (the secondary ossification center) due to contraction of the quadriceps muscle	• Common in participants of sports involving running and jumping • Common in adolescents following a rapid growth spurt
Popliteal synovial cyst (Baker's cyst)	• Enlargement of the gastrocnemius-semimembranosus bursa in the popliteal fossa	• Multifactorial (eg. trauma, coexistent, joint disease)	• Common in children and adults
Medial tibial stress syndrome (shin splints)	• Diffuse pain along the anterior aspect of the tibia (shinbone)	• Bone resorption > bone formation	• Common in runners
Compartment syndrome	• Increased pressure within a fascial compartment of a limb that compromises circulation	• Long bone fractures • Reperfusion injury • Animal venom	• Presents with pain out of proportion to findings and pain with passive stretching of the associated muscles • Motor deficits are a late finding (sign of irreversible damage)

Table 3.6.13 - Other conditions of the knee and leg

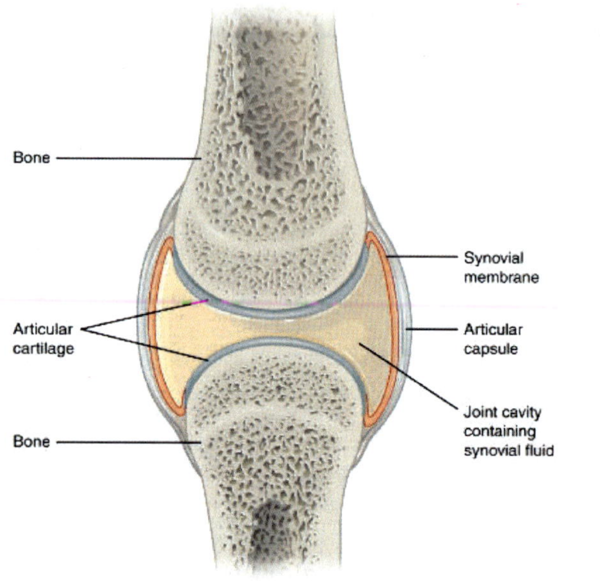

Figure 3.6.50 - The synovium

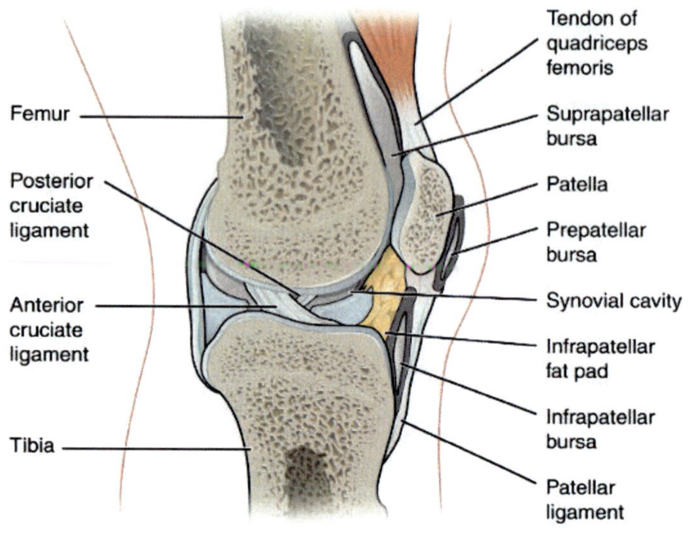

Figure 3.6.51 - Bursae of the knee

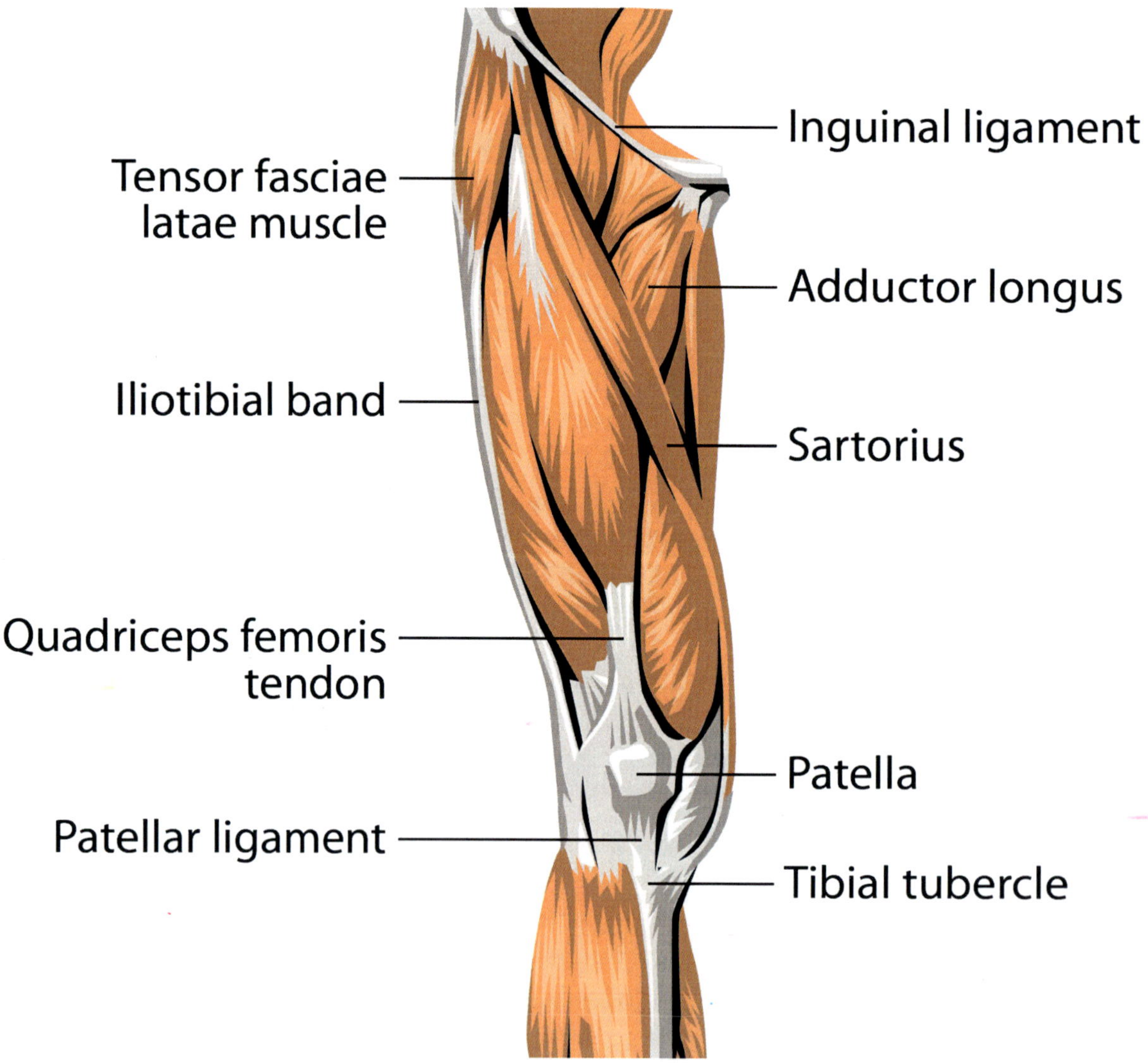

Figure 3.6.52 - Anterior view of the leg

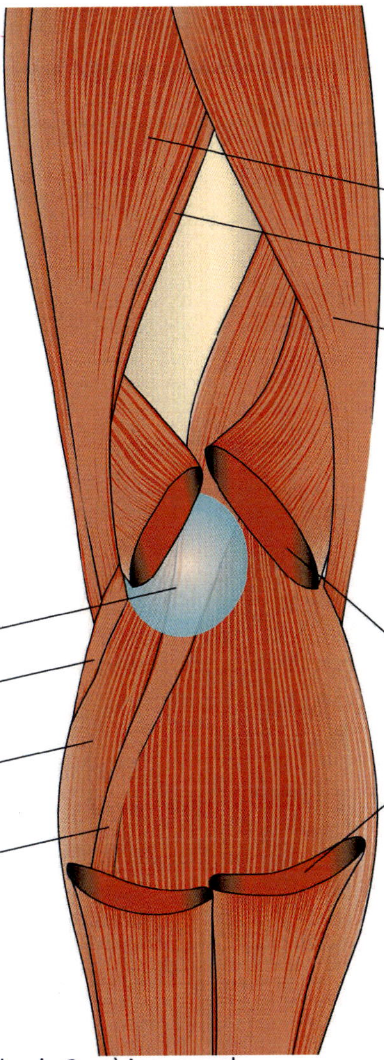

Figure 3.6.53 -Popliteal Synovial Cyst (Baker's Cyst) is named

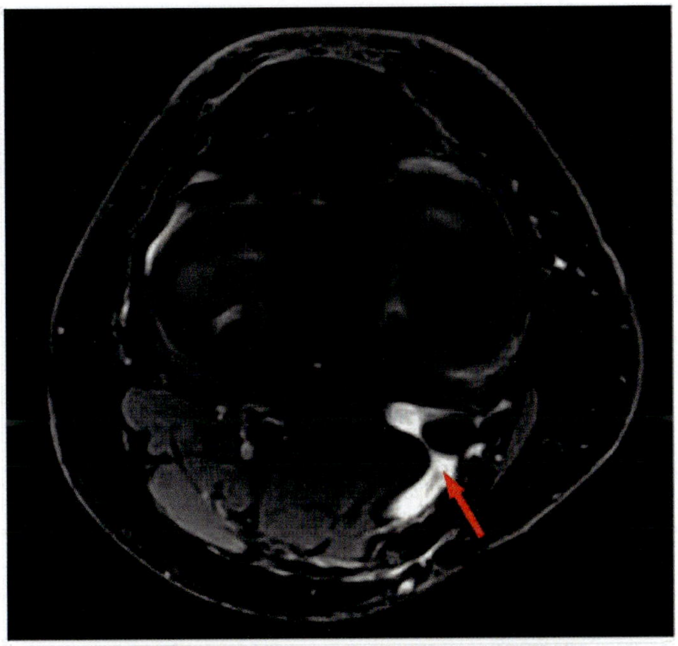

Figure 3.6.5 - MRI of a popliteal synovial cyst

REVIEW QUESTIONS

1. A 21-year-old male comes to the office due to knee pain which started 2 days ago. He is a missionary for his church and prays on his knees multiple times a day. Physical examination reveals no warmth, swelling, or erythema, but there is tenderness over the anterior aspect of the knee on palpation. Which of the following is the most likely diagnosis?

   A) Patellar fracture
   B) Osgood-Schlatter disease
   C) Popliteal synovial cyst
   D) Prepatellar bursitis
   E) Septic arthritis

- **Correct answer is D**
- **The patient prays on his knees multiple times a day (repetitive pressure) → inflammation of the prepatellar bursa → prepatellar bursitis**
- **A is incorrect - the patient reports no history of trauma**
- **B is incorrect - this is much more likely in an adolescent who recently underwent a rapid growth spurt or someone involved in aggressive sports activities**
- **C is incorrect - this typically presents with pain on the posterior aspect of the leg - not the anterior aspect of the knee**
- **E is incorrect - he has no warmth or swelling which is much more common in septic arthritis**

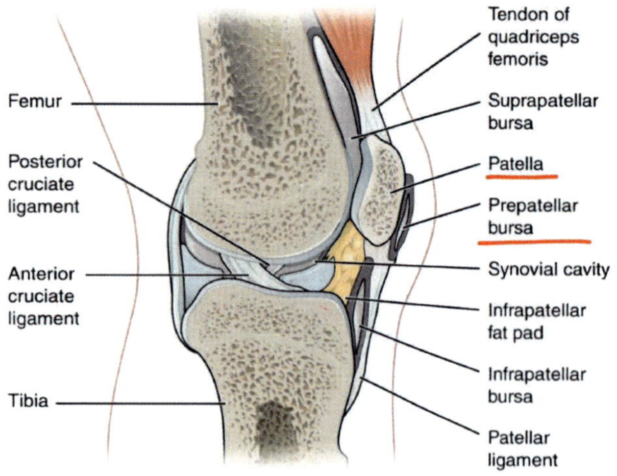

Section XI - Ankle and Foot

I. Ankle sprains

A. The lateral ligaments are weaker than the medial ligaments

B. The anterior talofibular ligament (ATFL) is most commonly injured

C. Often occurs following inversion of a plantar-flexed foot

D. Presents with pain and bruising near the anterolateral region of the ankle

E. The anterior inferior tibiofibular ligament is less commonly injured and presents with pain more proximally

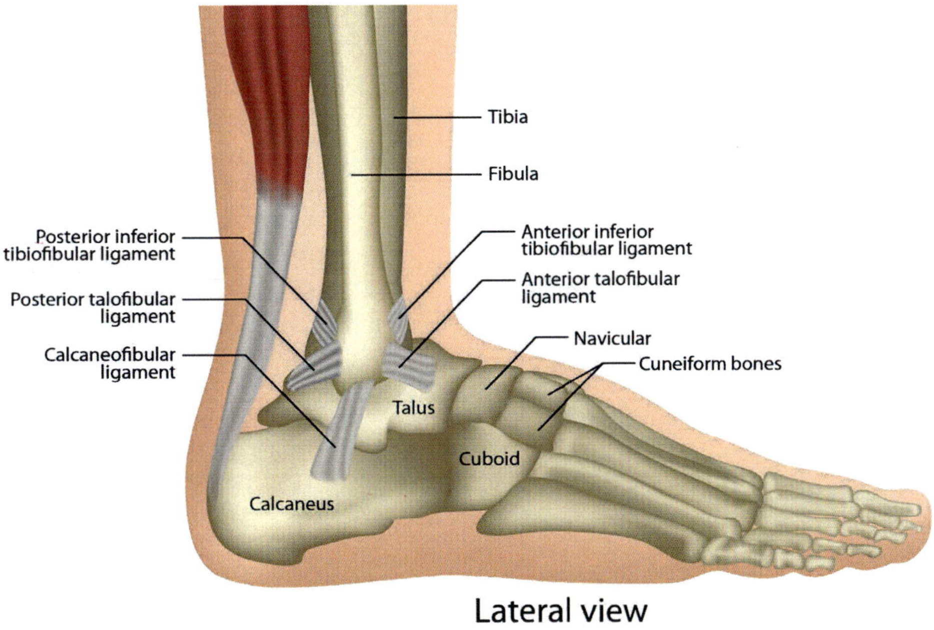

Figure 3.6.55 - Lateral view of the ankle

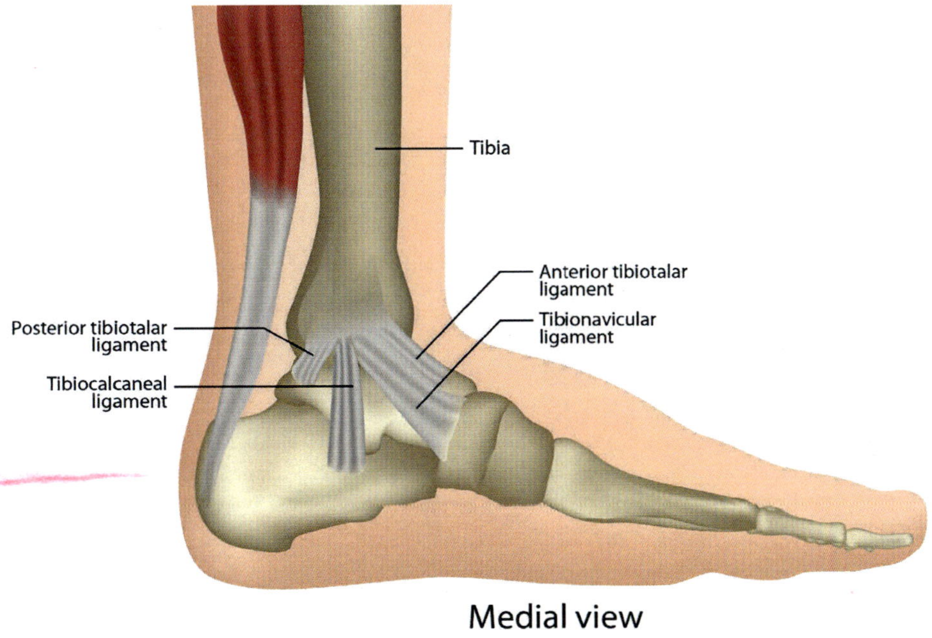

Figure 3.6.56 - Medial view of the ankle

II. Plantar fasciitis

A. Due to inflammation of the plantar aponeurosis

B. Unclear etiology (possibly due to a biomechanical abnormality)

C. Pain along the heel of the foot

D. Common in runners

E. Pain is worse with the first few steps after a period of inactivity

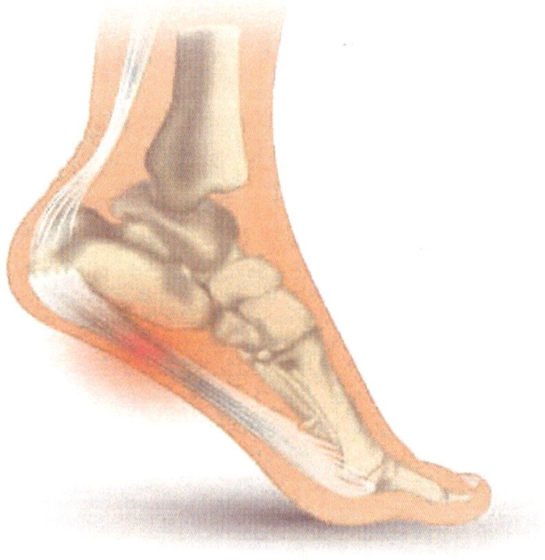

Figure 3.6.57 - Inflammation of the plantar aponeurosis

REVIEW QUESTIONS ?

1. A 24-year-old male is brought to the office after an ankle injury during a basketball game. He was running across the court when he twisted his left ankle inward. Physical examination reveals pain and bruising along the lateral aspect of the ankle joint. Which of the following structures is most likely injured?

A) Anterior tibiotalar ligament
B) Tibionavicular ligament
C) Anterior talofibular ligament
D) Posterior tibiotalar ligament
E) Tibiocalcaneal ligament

- **Correct answer is C**
- **The patient twisted his left ankle inward (ankle inversion) → pain along the lateral aspect of the ankle → ATFL injury (most common ankle injury)**
- **A, B, D, and E are all medial ankle ligaments which are less common and would present with pain along the medial aspect of the ankle joint**

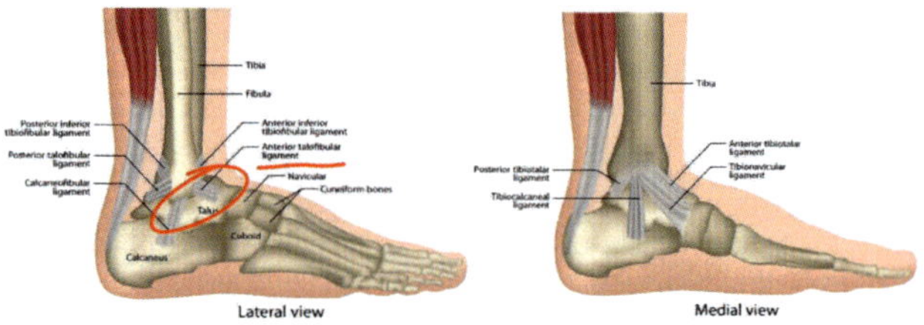

TABLES & FIGURES

INDEX